# Reflux and Heartburn

## The New Self-Help

# Jessica Madge

Coyote Digital Books

Cover design by John Amy

ISBN: 978-0-9574951-5-9

# Contents

*Introduction*

| | | |
|---|---|---|
| Chapter 1 | Symptoms and sufferers | 2 |
| Chapter 2 | Why reflux happens | 5 |
| Chapter 3 | Words of warning | 29 |
| Chapter 4 | Self Help Strategies | 39 |
| Chapter 5 | Strengthen your diaphragm | 44 |
| Chapter 6 | Reduce pressure | 61 |
| Chapter 7 | Work with gravity | 82 |
| Chapter 8 | Avoid irritants | 90 |
| Chapter 9 | Reduce stomach activity | 95 |
| Chapter 10 | Medicines and Self-help | 98 |
| Chapter 11 | How to help yourself | 111 |
| Appendix – | How the digestive system works | 117 |
| References | | 121 |
| Information sources on the Internet | | 125 |
| Also by Jessica Madge | | 127 |

# Introduction

I couple of years ago I developed acid reflux and I remembered that my mother suffered from life-long indigestion. Was this going to be a problem for the rest of *my* life?

Reflux is a very common medical problem and it's a miserable one. You suffer unpleasant burning sensations, an unwanted sour taste in your mouth or maybe even a nasty pain in your chest. Difficulty swallowing can make you conscious of every mouthful, so you eat cautiously, taking small mouthfuls and sipping water to help your food go down. People tell you to cut out a long list of foods. You stop enjoying your meals. And when you go to bed that burning in your chest keeps you awake or disturbs your sleep. Your symptoms prevent you from relaxing and enjoying life to the full.

My doctor immediately offered me acid-blocking medicine. But before I'd collected the prescription, someone suggested that reflux is a mechanical problem and that I had the knowledge to tackle it without drugs. Ten minutes spent with an anatomy textbook was a revelation. It seemed that it's not the amount of acid, or the strength of the acid that's the core of the problem. Instead, it's a "design flaw" at the top of the stomach. There's a natural anti-reflux barrier there, but it's not a strong one. This built-in weakness leaves us vulnerable to reflux.

So I began my personal search for physical solutions rather than chemical ones. Along the way I discovered many things you can do to minimise reflux, practical self-help techniques that are easy to do and don't cost a penny.

A few months later my symptoms were well controlled and I now only require an occasional antacid pill. My hope is that I will never have to depend on acid-blocking prescription drugs.

The approach outlined in this book will equip you to help yourself and manage with minimal aid from doctors, drugs or alternative practitioners. Help from doctors undoubtedly does have an important role in the management of reflux, as discussed in Chapters 2 and 10, but if you are looking for advice about anti-acid diets or herbs, you won't find it on these pages. If you sincerely want to help yourself or you just want to consider some new options, this book is for you.

Just to expand on my background a little, I studied Biology and Psychology at university then qualified to teach secondary school Biology. I taught for a few years, including lots of Human Biology courses. I also worked as an antenatal teacher, which involved extensive reading of medical books and a detailed study of breathing and relaxation techniques. After leaving school teaching I completed a master's degree by research and taught psychology to nurses on post-graduate courses in a university. Later I practised, studied and taught yoga. These aspects of my experience came together in the writing of this book.

It's aimed at the general reader and I've tried to reflect this in the style of writing. I've also tried to keep medical jargon to a minimum, but sometimes I have chosen a more medical word, "oesophagus" rather than "gullet", and "abdomen" instead of "tummy" or "belly", for instance. I've included a few diagrams and also kept them simple to meet the needs of ebook readers, who may be reading on small screens. Some readers may like to follow up in more detail, so I've included some key references at the back of the book.

I'd like to thank my son Toby, chiropractor and anatomy expert for the comment that steered me towards his shelf of anatomy books two years ago. Also my thanks to a group of friends who acted as proof-readers and critics. And last, but not least, a very big thank you to another friend, a retired gastrointestinal surgeon, who made many helpful comments and suggestions. Any remaining errors are my own

# Chapter 1

# Symptoms and Sufferers

Reflux is a common medical condition, usually minor, with far too many names and a confusing range of symptoms. It's known as: heartburn, acid reflux, gastric reflux, Gastro-Oesophageal Reflux Disease, GORD, Gastro-Esophageal Reflux Disease (The American spelling), GERD, GERS (gastro-esophageal reflux symptoms), acid regurgitation and acid indigestion to mention the most common.

In this book I'm going to stick to the word "reflux".

The medical profession has focussed on acid-blocking drugs and surgical techniques. But the drugs are not recommended for long-term continuous consumption and surgery is too drastic a solution for mild and moderate cases of reflux.

There is plenty of advice for those who suffer: avoid a long list of foods; eat small meals; prop up the head of your bed and so on. But much of this advice is general and aimed at all those suffering from "indigestion". Little of this advice has been scientifically tested and some of it is downright contradictory. A fresh look at the self-management of reflux is long overdue.

This book looks at the mechanics of reflux: what's going wrong, what can make it worse and how can you learn to control your symptoms?

It's a condition that varies a lot between individuals. There's no set pattern. Some people have occasional, mild symptoms while others have daily discomfort. A few have severe symptoms with a lot of pain. Some people have just one symptom, some have several and the pattern of symptoms can change over time.

The symptoms include:

- Burning sensations in throat, chest or back

- Acid coming back into mouth

- Discomfort on swallowing

- Pain or discomfort in chest or back

- Difficulty swallowing

- Hoarse voice

- Cough or wheezing

If you've started reading this, reflux is probably having an impact on your quality of life. It's uncomfortable. It can distract you from your work, spoil your leisure time and disrupt your sleep. It can also ruin your enjoyment of food. In the long-term, if not controlled, it can cause more serious health problems, (see Chapter 3)

But mostly it's just an uncomfortable nuisance that you would like to eliminate.

**What causes reflux?**

The symptoms of reflux are caused by acid flowing backwards from your stomach. It may gush up into your mouth or just seep upwards in tiny quantities.

Reflux is sometimes referred to as a kind of indigestion (or dyspepsia) but it's not a problem with digestion. Neither is it caused by too much acid in the stomach. It's a mechanical failure resulting from a weakness in the muscles at the top of your stomach. This weakness is often made worse by the way we use (or misuse) our bodies. In some of us there is also a bit of internal damage, known as hiatus hernia, which is contributing to the problem.

**Who gets reflux and why?**

**Babies.** Many of them regurgitate, "spit up" or "posset" regularly because the closure at the top of a baby's stomach is very weak. They tend to grow out of it as they get stronger and more active. It used to be thought harmless but these days many doctors think that some (the ones that are restless and crying) are suffering from discomfort, just like adults.

**Older adults.** Reflux becomes more and more common with age. As we get older we may become less active, all our muscles tend to get weaker and our bodies change in other ways. Hiatus hernia (explained in Chapter 2) is also increasingly common with age and this may contribute to the problem in some cases.

**Pregnant women.** The baby leaves less room for the stomach, squashing it and causing acid backflow. Pregnancy hormones also have a relaxing effect on some parts of the body and may affect the opening at the top of the stomach.

**People who are overweight**. Fat around the waist has a similar effect to pregnancy, putting pressure on the stomach.

**People who live in wealthy countries.** It's estimated that between 10% and 30% of adults in richer countries suffer from reflux regularly, compared to less than 10% in poorer ones. We don't know the reason for this but sedentary lifestyles and obesity may be to blame for the difference. There is some evidence that the incidence is increasing in western countries.

**People on prescription drugs**. Some medicines increase the risk of reflux.

**Smokers.** Reflux seems to be more common in smokers. You only have to look at the deeply lined faces of long-term smokers (compared to non-smokers of the same age) to see that smoking has a damaging effect on tissues throughout the body.

**People with certain medical conditions.** Diabetes, for instance, can slow down the emptying of the stomach, which can contribute to reflux. A poorly-functioning stomach exit valve can have the same effect. This condition is known as pyloric stenosis.

This book will explain how to strengthen the muscles that prevent backflow from your stomach. It will also explain how to work with your body to reduce pressure on your stomach and control your symptoms.

If you have fairly mild reflux, the advice in this book will enable you to keep it under control. For more severe cases, a realistic aim would be to reduce your symptoms and cut down on medication. The information in this book will also help you to make informed decisions about medication or surgery.

## How is the book structured?

In the next chapter there is a quick tour of the relevant parts of the body and an explanation of how a weakness at the top of your stomach can cause reflux. Chapter 3 goes on to explain some of the serious long-term complications of reflux and discusses different kinds of help and advice.

Chapters 4 to 9 outline a fresh approach to self-help for reflux sufferers, using physical solutions to address this mechanical problem.

I will explain some simple exercises that will help you to control your symptoms. Most of the exercises can be done anywhere, whenever you have a few minutes to spare. You will also discover how bending, lifting and constipation can contribute to your problem and how you can re-train your body to avoid putting pressure on your stomach.

There will also be suggestions about how you could adjust your lifestyle, and help your symptoms to calm down as quickly as possible.

Chapter 10 covers the medicines used for reflux and how these can be used alongside self-help.

Self-help is not a magic wand. It means taking the initiative, adapting your habits and changing your lifestyle. These require determination. But the incentive is strong – if you adapt the way you use your body the reward is a more comfortable life without the frequent discomfort that reflux can cause.

# Chapter 2

# Why reflux happens

In this chapter I'll be explaining how the mechanical workings of your stomach and parts of your body combine to cause reflux. This will help you to understand both your symptoms and the ways that the self-help techniques in this book work. If you'd like a quick recap of how the digestive system works you should read the appendix now but if you remember your school Biology lessons, read on.

**The oesophagus**

When you swallow a mouthful of food it passes into your oesophagus, a flexible tube, a couple of centimetres wide and about 25cms long. It starts at the back of your throat and goes straight down behind your larynx (voicebox) and windpipe.

The windpipe is a wide tube, held open by rings of cartilage. Its top end is widened and forms the larynx. The oesophagus, on the other hand, is a soft tube that opens up when something passes through. Although it's shown as an open tube in the diagram, it's normally collapsed, with its inner walls touching each other. If you imagine a long tube of rubbery, cooked pasta, that will give you the idea.

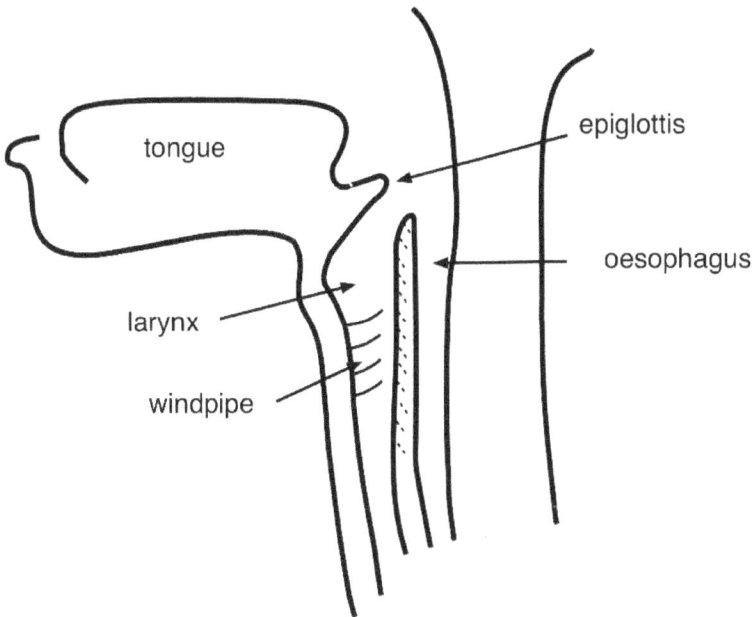

Its walls contain thin layers of muscle that squeeze to push food along, a process known as peristalsis. Every time you swallow, a wave of peristalsis passes down your oesophagus, pushing the food or drink downwards. The journey from mouth to stomach takes a few seconds. As your oesophagus descends through your chest, it passes behind your heart, turns left and joins your stomach at an angle.

If you are in a quiet place – maybe drinking some tea or water in bed – you may be able to hear your oesophagus working. Or rather, you can hear the fluid arriving in your stomach a few seconds after you have swallowed. It's a kind of gurgling, squirting sound as the muscles of the oesophagus push the liquid through the narrow opening at the top of your stomach. You might also be able to sense the passage of something very cold or hot as it travels downward. But generally speaking your oesophagus is not particularly sensitive – you only notice it when it is damaged or has been made sore and uncomfortable as a result of reflux.

**The stomach**

Some people use the word "stomach" to refer to the whole of their abdominal area, as in: "I've got stomach ache". But I'm using it in a more precise way. It's the large, hollow structure that lies at the end of your oesophagus, which acts as the first staging post in the process of digestion.

Your stomach sits on your left side, much higher than you might think. In fact it's tucked under the left side of your ribs. The top of it can be as high as nipple level. So if someone clutches their lower abdomen complaining of a "pain in my stomach", they're a long way off target. In the diagram you can see how it sits, more in the chest than the middle of the abdomen.

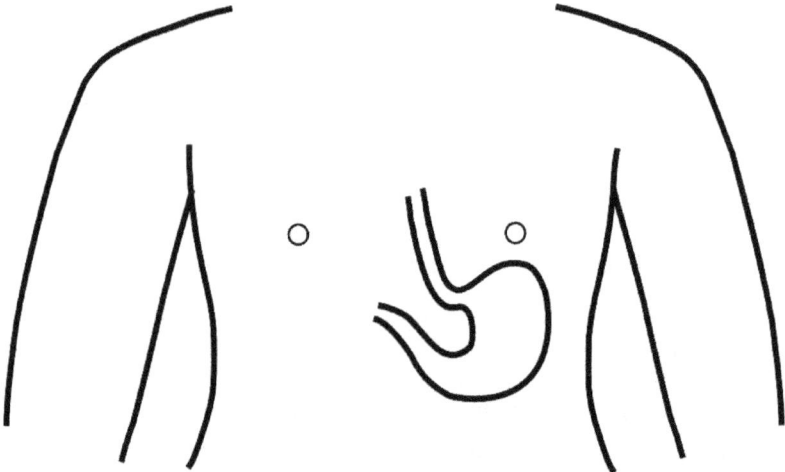

When it's empty it's shaped a bit like a sock, with the bulging heel at the top left hand side. But unlike a sock it has two openings - one near the top, where it's connected to the oesophagus, and the other at the right side, where it's joined to the small intestine (imagine a turned up toe of the sock with an opening at the toe end).

When you eat and drink, your stomach expands and becomes more bag-shaped. It can expand a lot. Think about the size of the largest meal you eat, on a feast day such as Christmas, Thanksgiving or Eid, including the drinks you consume with your food. As you eat, the glands in the wall of your stomach pour out gastric juices, which stretch it further. The bigger the meal, the more gastric juice will be produced. But that's not all. Your stomach probably contains some air as well, adding to its volume.

Once you've eaten, the food stays in your stomach for several hours because an important phase of digestion takes place there. (See Appendix for a recap on digestion). The exit from your stomach is controlled by a powerful sphincter valve known as the pyloric valve or pylorus. This strong, ring-doughnut-shaped muscle contracts around the tube leading from the stomach and keeps it closed until it receives a "relax" instruction from your nervous system. Then it opens to allow a little squirt of stomach contents to move on. The amount is small because the intestines are narrow and can only cope with a small amount at a time. Gradually the valve allows all the semi-digested food to pass on.

Gastric juice, secreted by the glands of the stomach contains hydrochloric acid. This acid is one of the body's defences because it can kill bacteria that cause food poisoning and dysentery. It also helps digestion by acting as a marinade, softening protein-based food like meat or fish. Gastric juice also contains an enzyme that starts to break down food. But the stomach doesn't soften or digest its own lining. It has a number of defences that prevent this.

As soon as the semi-digested food moves into the intestine, its acidity is rapidly neutralised by the secretions of the pancreas. This prevents acid damage to the wall of the intestine. However if any stomach contents back up into the oesophagus, there is less protection and the resulting acid burn is the cause of most of the pain and discomfort of reflux.

Gastric juice may be more damaging to the oesophagus than laboratory acid of identical strength. This is because it contains an enzyme, known as pepsin, which breaks down meat in the stomach. So we can assume that under the right circumstances it can also damage human flesh. No one really knows the extent to which pepsin contributes to reflux symptoms. For the purposes of this book, I will just refer to acid.

**The diaphragm**

The next body part to consider is the diaphragm, which forms part of the anti-reflux mechanism of the body. The centre of your body, your trunk, is divided into two compartments known as the chest cavity and the abdominal cavity. The word "cavity" sounds like an empty space, but both are completely filled with important organs. The heart, lungs and oesophagus are the main organs in your chest, while the liver, stomach, intestines and colon (bowel) are the biggest ones in your abdomen.

The chest cavity is surrounded by a cage of bones made up of the ribs, breastbone and spine. It's not a completely rigid cage as there are flexible joints at the front and back that allow a limited amount of rib movement.

The abdominal cavity is also bordered by the spine at the back, but otherwise it has soft walls, made up of sheets of abdominal muscle (known as "tummy muscles", "abs" or, these days, "core muscles").

These act like a corset, helping to flatten your abdomen and support your spine.

The dividing partition between the chest and the abdomen is a large sheet of muscle called the diaphragm. It's dome-shaped and stretches right across your rib cage from front to back and from side to side. Your heart sits just on top of it, with your spongy lungs wrapping snugly around the sides. Your stomach sits just below it. The next diagram shows how the stomach is tucked under the diaphragm.

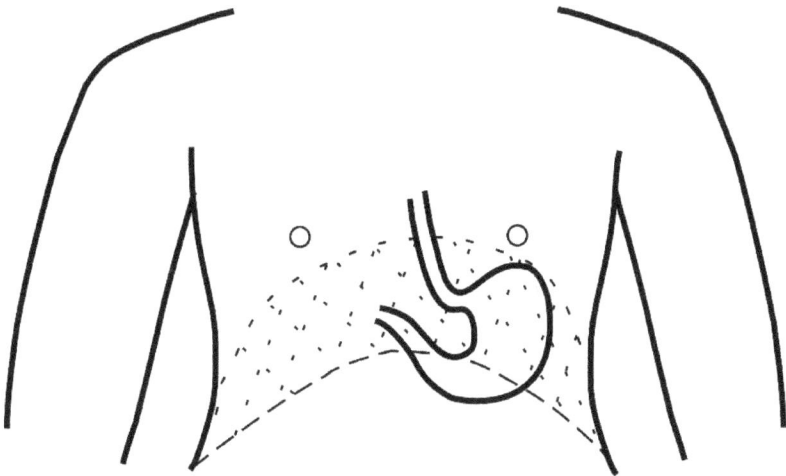

If you put a finger at the bottom of your breastbone, you'll get an idea where the front of your diaphragm is attached - to the inner side of the bone beneath your finger. The top of its dome is a little higher than this. If you trace around the edges of your ribs, you will get an idea of the position of its edges, which are lower at the sides and back than at the front. It's quite big – the size of a rather large, oval fruit bowl.

The diaphragm is a partition but it's certainly not a flat wall. It's more like a rounded tent with its highest point in the middle and its edges tethered much lower down. It's not a single muscle. Instead, it's made of several bands of muscle, layered in different directions. To envisage how your diaphragm is constructed out of these overlapping strips of muscle, imagine a circular trampoline made of several broad ribbons of rubber, stretched from one side to the other, in different directions and overlapping each other.

The diaphragm plays a part in preventing reflux but it is, of course, your main breathing muscle. When you breathe in, its muscle fibres are contracting. This makes it tighten, flatten and move down, pressing on your stomach and other abdominal organs. When you are breathing lightly it moves up and down a mere two or three centimetres but when you breathe very deeply it may move as much as eight or ten centimetres.

The downward movement of your diaphragm makes your chest cavity larger. This reduces pressure inside your chest, which has the effect of drawing air into your lungs. When you breathe out, your diaphragm relaxes, softens and rises upwards, pressing gently on your lungs and causing the air to flow out.

There are lots of smaller breathing muscles between your ribs, known as intercostal muscles. When they contract, your ribs swing slightly outwards and upwards, helping to make your chest cavity bigger. But your diaphragm, which is much more powerful than the intercostals, is the primary breathing muscle.

The main job of the diaphragm is to maintain a steady supply of oxygen to the body, and to get rid of carbon dioxide. But it does a number of other things:

- Responds to additional oxygen demands during exercise
- Plays a part in sneezing, yawning, coughing and choking

- Contributes to vomiting by lurching downwards

- Moves in a characteristic way when you sigh, laugh, cry or gasp with fear or pain

- Causes hiccups when it twitches

Your diaphragm is a special muscle because, like the heart, it keeps you alive and keeps working without the need to think about it. A primitive part of your brain controls it, just as it does in all mammals. But what makes it different from the heart is that it's also closely connected to your conscious brain - the part that can choose, voluntarily, how and when a muscle moves.

This complex control of the diaphragm makes human speech possible and is useful in other ways as well, for instance:

- You can control your breath to blow out candles, sniff a rose, play a trumpet or scream at your team in a sports event

- Trained public speakers, actors and singers can control their breathing and so manage the way they use their voices

- You can hold your breath to swim underwater or avoid inhaling smoke

The important point for us is that this dual control of the diaphragm means you can exercise and strengthen your diaphragm to help it control your reflux. I'll be explaining why this works in this chapter and how you can do it in Chapter 5.

**The lower oesophageal sphincter**

You would think, perhaps, that gravity would keep food inside your stomach. But you might decide to lie down after eating or even stand on your head, so your body needs a way to prevent backflow. Even if you remain upright, the anti-reflux mechanism must work efficiently because the stomach is very active. When it's digesting a meal its muscular walls squeeze strongly in order to mix food with gastric juice. These contractions have the potential to push stomach contents backwards through a weak inlet valve. And the inlet is naturally weak.

If you've been reading other material about reflux you may have come across mention of the Lower Oesophageal Sphincter. It's commonly referred to as the LOS or the LES (based on the American spelling - esophagus).

You may have read that a weakness in the LOS causes reflux. This sounds completely reasonable but many writers go on to imply that the LOS is a muscular structure at the end of the oesophagus. That's what a sphincter normally is, a doughnut shaped muscle that acts like a valve, opening and closing a tube. If you are having trouble imagining how a sphincter works, imagine someone grasping around the outside of a soft tube with a fist, which usually grips tightly but occasionally relaxes. Classic examples of sphincters can be found at the outlet of the stomach, in the urethra and in the anus.

However, if you peer at anatomical diagrams of the stomach or photographs of dissected stomachs, there is no visible sphincter at the end of the oesophagus. At the outlet of the stomach you can see the thick, doughnut ring of the sphincter. But at the top end, nothing is visible. All that can be seen are thin layers of muscle similar to those that bring about peristalsis. So there is no strong, fist-like grip around this important junction, just a rather weak muscular squeezing effect from the walls at the bottom of the oesophagus. On detailed microscopic examination of this part of the oesophagus it is possible see that the thin layer of muscle is adapted to maintaining a gentle squeeze most of the time. This has been described as a sphincter, but it is certainly not a very powerful one compared to the stomach's outlet valve.

The LOS can be imagined more like the cuff on the sleeve of a knitted garment - a slightly more elastic section at the end of a long tube.

The important point that is often left out is this: the weak closure of the stomach entrance gets some help from the diaphragm, because it pinches the bottom of the oesophagus and helps to keep it closed. This help is obviously stronger when the diaphragm is tightening as you breathe in and weaker as you breathe out. It is possible that this continuous gentle rhythm helps the oesophagus to clear acid.

Some experts do recognise the role of the diaphragm and talk about the LOS having two parts, the inner LOS – the muscles in the wall of the lower oesophagus and the outer LOS – the pinching action of the diaphragm. The two work together to act as part of the body's anti-reflux barrier that prevents stomach contents from leaking up the oesophagus. But the strength of the LOS is much less than the strength of the stomach exit valve – it is, therefore, the weak spot if there is any undue pressure on the stomach.

Some men find it difficult to buy shirts with sleeves that are short enough for them. They solve this by using elasticated arm-bands, worn above the elbow. These grip the sleeve and keep it in place so the cuffs don't slide down too far. This is similar to the way the diaphragm grips around the oesophagus. So if you imagine the bottom of the oesophagus as an elasticated sleeve with one of those arm bands around the outside, that would be a model of how the oesophagus is kept closed. In the diagram you can see the arrangement I am describing.

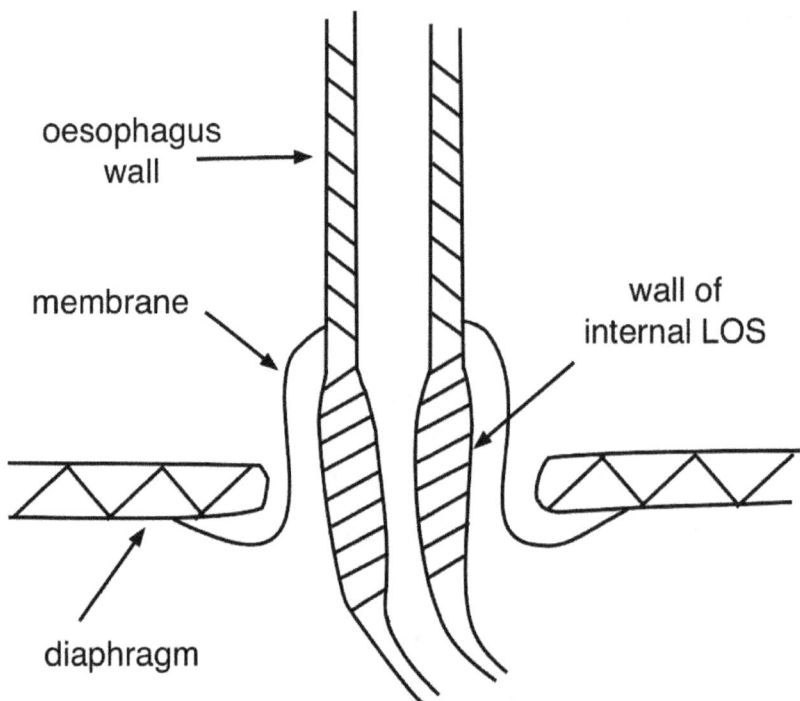

oesophagus wall

membrane

wall of internal LOS

diaphragm

This information about the diaphragm is very useful to reflux sufferers. You have no control over the muscles in the walls of your oesophagus but you do have control of your diaphragm and you can strengthen it with exercises and so reduce your symptoms of reflux. This will be covered in Chapter 5.

There is also an upper oesophageal sphincter, just behind the larynx. This tends to stop regurgitated fluid from entering the mouth but this does not protect the oesophagus from reflux. If there is frequent gushing of acid into the back of your mouth, or mouthfuls of reflux at night, this would indicate that you have significant weakness at both ends of your oesophagus and need to have a serious talk with your doctor (see Chapters 3 and 10).

## The hiatus

Hiatus means a pause and it's the term used for the place where the oesophagus passes through the diaphragm and where the diaphragm squeezes the oesophagus. It's like a chicane on a motor racing track. If you think of that trampoline made of rubber strips and then imagine a soft-walled hosepipe pushed between the strips you can envisage how the tension of the rubber would tend to have a squeezing action on the pipe.

The pinch point must not be too tight, because food has to pass into the stomach but it needs to be tight enough to help prevent backflow from the stomach.

The hiatus is a clever bit of natural engineering and to prevent the oesophagus sliding about there has to be something anchoring it to the diaphragm. The connection is provided by a circular ligament, which is shown in the diagram, above. Ligaments are elastic attachments between two moving body parts. Some, like the ones in the knee, are tough sinews. But this one is a rather flimsy circle of tissue, anchoring the oesophagus to the diaphragm. It has to be very flexible, otherwise it could not cope with all the activity that is going on:

- Movement of the oesophagus during peristalsis
- Up and down movement of diaphragm
- The stomach contracting strongly, nearby
- Constantly changing pressure on the two sides of the hiatus

## Hiatus hernia

Hernia is a term used by doctors when internal organs bulge through a weakness in a layer of muscle. Common sites are the groin and umbilicus. The term hiatus hernia (or hiatal hernia) refers to a bulging through the diaphragm, at the hiatus. This bulging results from a hiatus that has been weakened and widened and a ligament that has been stretched. The bulge could involve the short section of the oesophagus that normally lies below the diaphragm, or it could, in worse cases, include part of the stomach.

A really bad hiatus hernia involves a big gap in the diaphragm and needs surgery to correct it. Occasionally, when the diaphragm has not formed properly, a baby is born with such a gap. This is a known as a congenital hiatus hernia.

The most common type in adults is known as "sliding hiatus hernia", which occurs when the bottom end of the oesophagus slides back up through the hiatus. Think of it as being like a sleeve that is pushed up your arm. It's easy to imagine how symptoms could vary from day to day. One day the bottom of your oesophagus is in its correct position and other days it's a bit wrinkled up. It's like a man trying to keep his shirt-sleeves in place with an unreliable arm band.

In a bigger hernia part of the stomach is bulging through the hiatus into the chest. The diagram on the next page shows this hernia with a lot of stretching at the hiatus. The other kind of diaphragmatic hernia, and the less common, is when a bubble of stomach wall pushes up through a weak spot somewhere else in the diaphragm. This is sometimes referred to as a "rolling" diaphragmatic hernia. It is not associated with reflux.

It's estimated that as many as one-third of people over 50 have a hiatus hernia – something doctors could see if they investigated. But not all these people have symptoms. Even when a doctor looks down the oesophagus with an endoscope (a fine fibre-optic instrument), the area is moving around, making hernias tricky to diagnose. A barium meal X ray is sometimes used to get a more accurate picture.

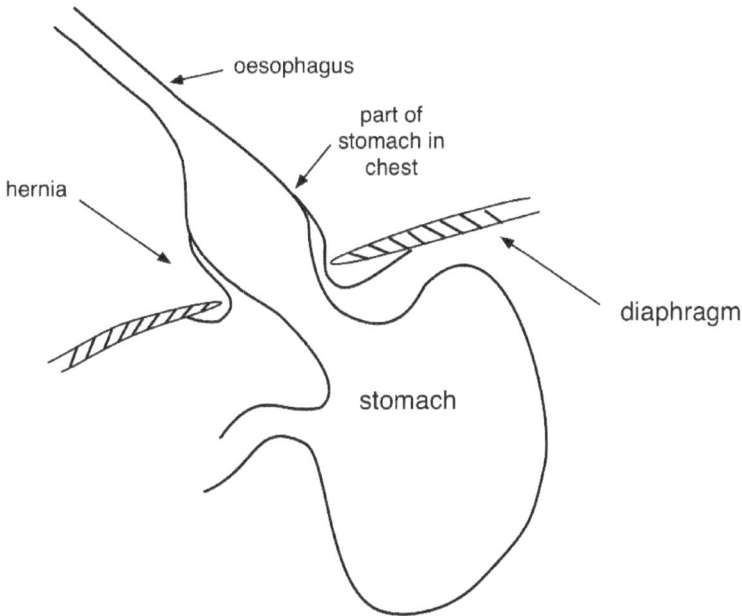

oesophagus

part of
stomach in
chest

hernia

diaphragm

stomach

You may be wondering what causes a typical hiatus hernia? How and
why does the hiatus become wider and how is the ligament stretched?
We can only guess, but it could be that violent movement of the
diaphragm could have caused it during sneezing, coughing or vomiting.
Another possibility is too much pressure from below, resulting from
pregnancy, too much fat in the abdomen or straining. An oesophagus that
has been damaged due to long-term reflux can also, eventually, become
scarred and shortened and may tend to tug the stomach upwards through
the weak area.

### Have I got reflux or a hernia?

The symptoms of hiatus hernia are highly variable so even your doctor
might not be able to tell (without tests) whether you have straightforward

reflux or reflux associated with a hernia. Hiatus hernia was, at one time, seen as *the* cause of reflux. Now, it is seen as one of several factors that can *predispose* someone to reflux.

One suggestion as to why a hiatus hernia might increase reflux is that when it slides, the squeezing at the hiatus is no longer lined up with the area where the oesophagus tends to squeeze itself shut. Another is that when it moves upwards, the angle between oesophagus and the stomach straightens out and this makes it easier for acid to escape. The exact nature of the mechanical failure is hard (or maybe impossible) to investigate.

The three common types of hernia – at the groin, at the umbilicus and at the hiatus all take place at weak spots in the walls of the abdominal cavity. Once a small amount of damage has occurred at one of these weak spots there's potential for the hernia to get bigger. Imagine a small hole in a paper bag. If you keep pushing your finger through it, the hole will get wider and wider. So it is important, if you seem to have a weakness in the area, to avoid things that might make any tendency to hernia worsen. There will be some suggestions about how to do this in Chapter 6 and 7.

**Why are there so many symptoms relating to reflux?**

Researchers have discovered that the LOS doesn't maintain a steady pressure. There is the continuous rhythmic squeezing of the diaphragm of course and they have also observed what they call "transient relaxations" of the LOS when the normal squeezing effect of the walls relaxes, allowing acid to flow backwards for a few moments. These relaxations happen all the time in healthy people and they cause a normal, harmless level of reflux. An obvious example is when you burp, but other less obvious relaxations also happen. In some people backflow happens more frequently, or the acid stays in the oesophagus longer and they develop reflux symptoms. As in all parts of the body, there are individual differences in size and shape of the stomach and other organs and it could be that some people are just more physically susceptible to reflux than others.

The acid in the stomach is stronger than vinegar or lemon juice. If you got some lemon juice in your eye it would sting badly and your eye would quickly redden. If this happened repeatedly during the day, you'd have a very sore eye by bed-time. So you can imagine that over-exposure of the lining of the oesophagus to a fairly strong acid could make it sore. Reflux symptoms may be caused by a few prolonged, or many, repeated backflows during the day. One way of understanding this is to imagine you pass your hand through a candle flame. If you do it quickly you won't get burned but if you keep your hand in the flame too long, or you keep putting it back and fore repeatedly, you will.

When acid stays in a healthy stomach it causes no harm and no inflammation. The stomach lining has its own defences to protect it. But the lining of the oesophagus is not so well protected and acid can cause damage and a sore, inflamed lining. Doctors call this oesophagitis. This just means inflammation of the oesophagus.

Inflammation is the immune system's reaction to tissue damage. It's the work of the emergency division of the immune system that causes tiny blood vessels to dilate and millions of extra immune cells (white blood cells) rush to the area. These, in turn, produce billions of powerful immune molecules (known as cytokines). The side effects of all this are swelling, redness and pain. This is quite separate from the slower work that the adaptive division of the immune system does by developing antibodies and long-term immunity to individual diseases. (To learn more about the immune system see my first book – details at the end of this one).

Inflammation is a wonderful thing – it will usually prevent a serious bacterial infection if you cut yourself. The trouble is that it doesn't just occur when you have a wound - other kinds of tissue damage can set it off, such as a sprained ankle, a burn or acid damage.

An acid-burned, inflamed oesophagus is the cause of many of the symptoms of reflux. It could just cause a mild burning or it could be sharp pain or burning sensation in the chest. For some people the pain can be agonising. It can even be mistaken for angina or a heart attack (remember the oesophagus sits immediately behind the heart). It may be made worse by bending forward, lying down or straining (as in lifting something heavy or straining on the toilet).

Once your oesophagus has got damaged and inflamed it will take some time to settle – the length of time depends on the amount of damage. It's not got a great blood supply so it probably won't heal as quickly as the lining of your mouth.

If prolonged inflammation occurs anywhere in the body it tends to cause collateral damage. The chemicals of inflammation are very powerful, they can kill bacteria and they can, ultimately, damage body cells. This is why long-term inflammation of the oesophagus can cause further problems (see Chapter 3).

**What is "silent reflux"?**

Another group of symptoms relate to the larynx and windpipe: hoarse voice, cough and wheezing. This set of symptoms is sometimes referred to as "silent reflux" because it may occur in the absence of other reflux symptoms. In other people these larynx-related symptoms occur alongside other symptoms. It's obviously important that food and drink don't go down your windpipe. To prevent this there is a small flap called the epiglottis that closes over the top of the windpipe every time you swallow.

If food gets into your windpipe and "goes down the wrong way" your body reacts violently by coughing. The larynx and windpipe are extremely sensitive to anything other than air entering them because the lungs are very delicate. Just a whiff of smoke or a drop of water is all it takes to trigger coughing.

It's easy to imagine that tiny drops of stomach acid, coming up into the larynx frequently, could cause problems. The amount of acid must be very small, or it would cause choking.

Doctors are not in total agreement about the diagnosis "silent reflux". If someone has an inflamed or irritated larynx and symptoms are persisting, a course of acid-blocking drugs is often prescribed. Sometimes this works, in which case everyone concludes that reflux was the cause of the problems, but in some cases the drugs don't work. It is still a bit of a mystery. The only way to be sure whether or not there is acid in the larynx is for a doctor to test it for acidity, using a tiny probe.

In the past, doctors tended to lay the blame for reflux on a single cause: over-indulgence of rich food; hiatus hernia; faulty LOS and so on. These days they see it as "multifactorial" with factors like obesity playing a part alongside the factors that cause poor closure at the top of the stomach. Later on in this book you will find out how to tackle some of these in order to bring your symptoms under control.

I hope that you have now got a clear picture of the way that a weak junction between the oesophagus and the stomach can cause such a variety of symptoms. In the next chapter, I will look at some of the medical complications that can arise from long-term reflux, explain when and why you should take advice from your doctor and discuss why you should be cautious about alternative medicine and health advice on the Internet.

# Chapter 3

# Words of Warning

It's good to be enthusiastic about self-help but, as with many things, a few basic facts and a bit of common sense are also important. There are times when reflux suffers need to decide if self-help is the best approach or whether it's time to see a doctor as well. This chapter covers some important information that will help you to make informed choices.

Firstly, it is important to be aware that long-term reflux can eventually cause permanent damage, which may, in turn, lead to much more serious conditions. So you shouldn't just put up with it on a long-term basis. The sooner you tackle the problem the less likely you are to suffer something more serious in the years to come.

Here are some of the things that are associated with long-term acid damage to the oesophagus:

**Erosive oesophagitis**

If you have persistent reflux you could develop ulceration of the oesophagus. In other words it has gone beyond simple inflammation and eroded away a layer of tissue. This is a serious condition that can cause bleeding and sharp pain. Your doctor will probably prescribe a course of acid-blocking medicine to help it to heal. You should take the full course. For further information on medicines see Chapter 10.

If you've ever had mouth ulcers you'll know they can take a time to heal. But erosive oesophagitis is potentially a lot more serious than a little mouth ulcer. You may also be referred for an endoscopic examination. The examining doctor will use a narrow, fibre-optic tube, to get a close-up view of your oesophagus to see exactly what is happening.

**Stricture**

Some sufferers have temporary difficulty swallowing (dysphagia) because exposure to acid has made the lining of the oesophagus inflamed and swollen or because a hiatus hernia is playing up. When this happens you feel you have to chew more thoroughly, eat more slowly and take sips of water to get a mouthful down.

Long-term acid damage can cause a more serious kind of dysphagia, known as "stricture", in other words scarring that has narrowed the oesophagus. This can cause permanent difficulty swallowing.

**Shortened oesophagus**

If your oesophagus is scarred by long-term reflux it can become shorter. This can tend to make a hiatus hernia worse by tugging the stomach upwards.

**Barrett's oesophagus**

This is a condition in which there are permanent changes to the cells that have been affected by exposure to stomach acid. You would only know about this if you had tests, as it has no symptoms. Once the changes to the cells have happened there is an increased risk of cancer developing, so it's often described as a pre-cancerous condition. According to Cancer

Research UK, between 1% and 5% of people with Barrett's go on to develop cancer of the oesophagus. So Barrett's is a warning sign not a diagnosis of cancer.

**Cancer of the oesophagus**

This cancer is on the increase but it is still not common. According to Cancer Research UK there are around 8,300 cases in the UK per year (as compared to over 40,000 per year for both lung cancer and bowel cancer). It's twice as common in men as it is in women and the same applies to erosive oesophagitis and Barrett's.

Reflux and long-term oesophagitis both increase your risk of cancer of the oesophagus, as do smoking and alcohol consumption. Obesity too increases the chances of developing this cancer, possibly due to a link between obesity and reflux. Eating a lot of meat that has been cooked at high temperatures may also increase the risk.

Bear in mind that reflux is just *one* possible cause of oesophageal cancer and that the disease usually takes years to develop. Like reflux, it has several possible causes that may interact over a number of years to create the disease. In other words, don't lose sleep worrying about cancer if you have had reflux for a few weeks. But problems with your oesophagus should not be shrugged off and ignored for years on end.

**Is it really reflux?**

The second thing you should be aware of is that there is a range of medical conditions that can produce symptoms similar to some of those caused by reflux. Abdominal pain and chest pain can be hard for doctors to diagnose.

The easiest way to find out if sharp pain is due to reflux or not is to stand up and have a good drink of water. This will wash away or dilute the acid in your oesophagus. If your pain eases, usually with a minute or so, then it is probably due to reflux.

*if you have bad pain in your chest that comes on suddenly and is not relieved by a glass of water (and you haven't had it checked by a doctor), you need urgent medical attention to ensure it is not a heart attack or other life-threatening event.*

Any cough, sore throat, hoarse voice, pain, swallowing problem or digestive change that goes on more than a couple of weeks should always be referred to your doctor because there are many conditions that can cause these symptoms.

Use your common sense. If you had a cold, then a cough, and it's gradually getting better, you don't need a doctor. But if you have a croaky or uncomfortable throat that doesn't seem related to a cold (or to shouting in a noisy social event) and it doesn't seem to be getting better after a couple of weeks, then see your doctor.

Stomach pain may be caused by inflammation of the stomach lining, known as gastritis. Regular consumption of anti-inflammatory drugs (such as aspirin or ibuprofen) is a known cause and so is over-consumption of alcohol.

The other common cause of gastritis is Helicobacter pylori, a very unusual bacterium that thrives in the stomach. It doesn't cause vomiting and diarrhoea. Instead it can cause long-term inflammation of the stomach lining. Stomach acid is a very hostile environment for most bacteria and the medical world took some convincing that H. pylori actually existed. It is now accepted as an important cause of gastritis, peptic ulcers (painful and potentially dangerous sores on the wall of the stomach and upper intestine) and some stomach cancers. If you are suffering from painful "indigestion" it could be that H. pylori related gastritis or an actual ulcer is the reason. The correct antibiotic can clear the infection if you take the full course.

Helicobacter is transmitted in saliva so if you are diagnosed, ask your doctor if your partner can have the simple test for it as well.

There are other conditions that could cause a range of "indigestion" symptoms. So if you are having symptoms on a regular basis, it's important to talk them through with your doctor. There are a few very rare conditions that can cause reflux but reflux is extremely common and most cases do not have any underlying medical problem.

The National Health Service advice website recommends that you should talk to your doctor if you have indigestion, reflux-like symptoms, or stomach pain *and* if any of these apply to you:

- You are 55 years old or over

- You've lost a lot of weight without meaning to

- You've experienced difficulty swallowing (dysphagia)

- You are suffering from persistent vomiting (lasting more than a day or so)

- You've been told that you are anaemic

- You have blood in your vomit

- You've noticed blood in your stools or tarry stools (a sign of bleeding)

- You have a lump in your stomach

In Chapter 10 there is an explanation of the various medicines that can be prescribed by your doctor.

## Can alternative medicine help?

My third note of caution is about consulting people who are not qualified doctors. Some people, if suffering from minor medical conditions, consult an alternative practitioner such as a naturopath, herbalist, acupuncturist or homeopath. Consultations with such practitioners are typically longer than doctors' appointments and patients might feel they are being listened to and supported.

I am highly sceptical about the wisdom of consulting such practitioners. They are not trained to spot serious medical conditions so you should not consult them to get a diagnosis. *It is, frankly, dangerous to rely on alternative practitioners for diagnosis.*

It is also dangerous to follow their advice instead of mainstream medicine if you have a life-threatening illness such as cancer or diabetes. They may offer complementary therapies, like massage, that make you feel better, but cannot cure diseases.

I am also concerned that many alternative practitioners seem to give generic dietary advice to their customers such as "give up dairy" and "give up gluten". If too many elements are excluded from your diet, you risk malnutrition or vitamin deficiencies. There are only a very few diseases in which particular foods must be avoided for sound medical reasons (gluten in cases of coeliac disease and sugar in diabetes being the main ones). The best person to advise on diet and medical conditions is a qualified dietitian (not a "nutritional therapist").

Alternative practitioners sometimes tell their clients that certain foods or diets can cure them. Neither individual foods nor special diets cure illnesses. They might help your to stay healthy and they might help your recover from illness but they are not cures. The only exceptions are vitamin deficiency diseases that are cured by consuming the missing vitamins. However there is very little evidence to support the taking of vitamin supplements by healthy people.

*The idea that a wide range of diseases, including cancer, can be cured by dietary methods is wrong and dangerous.*

Some alternative practitioners recommend herbs. Herbal medicines and supplements are not necessarily safe and can, like prescription drugs, cause dangerous side effects. Safe levels of intake, particularly long-term intake, are not known because the research has not been done.

You should not take herbal medicines alongside prescription medicines because harmful interactions can occur. These herb-drug interactions are not well researched. Herbs can also be contaminated if they do not come from a reputable source.

Homeopathy is completely safe because it contains no active ingredients whatsoever. This also means that, other than the placebo effect, the preparations are completely useless.

Sometimes the placebo effect, which may be induced by alternatives, can reduce the way people experience symptoms such as pain or nausea. But the placebo effect certainly cannot cure any actual diseases. Neither is it reliable – it can be observed to help some of the symptoms, in some of the people, some of the time.

Alternative practitioners are, generally speaking, not regulated (there may be exceptions that vary between countries) so that's another problem – there's no professional oversight so there's nobody to complain to if you are unhappy.

Consulting an alternative practitioner is not "self-help", it's hoping that someone else will fix your symptoms.

**Is the Internet a good source of help?**

My final caution is about looking for advice on-line.

If you search the Internet for medical advice and information you can find some that is good, lots that is bad and some that is downright ugly. There are many sites that are shop windows for "supplement" sales. Others are selling unproven procedures like "colonic irrigation" or fraudulent devices like "energy bracelets". Even worse, there are many sites promoting and selling fake cancer cures. If you think of a life-threatening disease and type its name into a search engine you will find many websites that seek to exploit people with a terminal prognosis.

Unfortunately, due to the international nature of the Web, it is impossible for individual governments to control misleading and fraudulent sites.

Unless you have some scientific training it is hard to sort through the sheer quantity of online advice and advertising. Sites selling supplements often cite small, preliminary studies (which may relate to cells in a dish, a one off study in laboratory mice or a poorly designed study with a few humans) and use them as a platform to trumpet the latest miracle remedy or food.

There is a list of some reputable sources of information at the back of the book and I recommend you start with these if you want to do some online research.

If you search the Internet, you may well find some individual alternative practitioners claiming they have *the* cure for reflux.

For example some claim that massage or manipulation over the left side of the abdomen enables them to "draw down" a hiatus hernia. This just might, possibly, be the case, but there is no reason to think that it will *stay* down after such a treatment. But it seems to me that the area involved is tucked well under the rib cage, and is therefore not accessible to the hands of a masseur. If you have a hernia, and if it could be drawn downwards, nothing is going to stop it sliding back up again later in the day.

I suggest that you do not waste money on this kind of procedure.

Another recommendation doing the rounds on the Internet is that drinking some warm water first thing in the morning and then bouncing up and down on your heels will "end your acid reflux problems". The idea is, presumably, that you jolt a hernia back down through your diaphragm. This seems to be one of those Internet myths that gets picked up and re-used on poor-quality websites. Why should warm water work better than a cup of tea? And why should your hernia stay down for the rest of the day, just because you have done a bit of bouncing in the morning?

If this technique works on a temporary basis, we should assume that drinking any fluid and then skipping, jumping off the bottom step of your staircase, bouncing on a trampoline or even going for a run, at any time of day, would all be equally effective.

Any approach that physically moves a hernia downwards can only be a temporary fix at best because it is not tackling the underlying causes of your problem.

**Summary of chapter:**

- Don't just tolerate reflux or indigestion for a long time

- Consult your doctor if you have indigestion symptoms that are regular or severe

- Stop and think carefully before spending money on alternatives

- Be very cautious when searching for health advice on the Internet and look for reputable sites

# Chapter 4

# Self-Help Strategies

Your digestive system is a bit like a factory production line. Raw materials go in at one end and pass along, going though various stages, each of with its own specialised engineering.

Imagine there's a rather temperamental valve near the beginning of a factory line. Every so often a red light flashes and there are clunky noises that get on everyone's nerves. The process still works and the engineers can't justify an expensive re-design so they nurse along the valve to minimise annoyance. Every day they add a little lubrication, tighten up a few nuts and fiddle with the settings. As long as they attend to it regularly, they can minimise the irritation it's causing and stop it getting worse.

Reflux is also a mechanical problem. In those of us who have a tendency to reflux, a "design flaw" means a valve that closes the stomach is not working perfectly. When you embark on self-help, it's a process of making adjustments to get the best out of this unreliable body part.

**The aims of self-help are:**

1. Minimise your reflux symptoms

2. Increase your comfort and enjoyment of life

3. Sleep more comfortably

4. If you have a hernia, try to avoid making it worse

5. Reduce your need for medication

The rest of this book covers five self-help principles. Each of them leads logically to things you can do on a daily basis to minimise your symptoms.

I've mentioned already that reflux happens to everyone to some extent but most people don't get symptoms. There is no single reason why some people get symptoms and some do not. It may be that some have many more reflux events in their day or that acid clears more slowly out of the oesophagus. It's also possible that in some people the oesophagus becomes more sensitive to acid over time.

But whatever the reasons, there are things we can all do to cut down the amount of reflux we're having.

The word indigestion (or dyspepsia if you are a doctor) is often used to cover the wide range of the symptoms produced by the stomach and oesophagus. The self-help advice that is offered is often generic, with the same advice given to all patients.

Some of this advice relates to food and drink that supposedly make symptoms worse. The list is quite long – high fat, high carbohydrate, chocolate, spices, coffee, peppermint, and so on. If you were to search on the Internet for half an hour you could extend this list considerably. However there is not a great deal of research into specific foods and whether or not they cause symptoms.

A 'systematic review' is an academic article in which the authors have gathered together all the scientific evidence they can find on a particular topic. They look at whether the original research has been conducted properly (e.g. was there a control group) and whether all the research results are in agreement or not. In a major review by medical researchers into whether dietary changes reduce reflux, the authors concluded that there is no strong evidence that altering any specific aspect of your diet will help. So despite doctors and many others advocating dietary changes there is no particular reason to think that giving up your favourite foods will help. However individuals do sometimes report that particular foods seem affect their symptoms. There will be further discussion of this in Chapters 8 and 9.

Smoking is also implicated in reflux by some studies but studies into *giving up* smoking don't all reach the same conclusions. Some seem to show improvement and some don't. It may be that smokers' coughs can cause hiatus hernia, in which case stopping smoking will not reverse the damage.

Where stronger evidence does exist, I've tried to include it at a relevant point.

There is a general lack of evidence into self-help measures to help control reflux and I cannot claim a strong evidence base for the suggestions in this book, but they are based on human anatomy, logic and common sense.

Many of them involve your making some small change to your daily habits. Each change takes time and a certain amount of focus and determination. So don't feel that you should tackle everything at once.

You can't expect to change lots of habits at the same time. There is some advice on making changes are the end of the book.

**The six areas of self-help that I've teased out are:**

**1. Strengthen your diaphragm** (Chapter 5)

By improving the strength and tone of your diaphragm you can improve its sphincter-like action and reduce backflow. I've drawn on my experience as an antenatal teacher and teacher of yoga to develop a graduated series of exercises that will strengthen your diaphragm and help it to perform its reflux-controlling duties. The key exercises can be done lying in bed or sitting in a chair.

**2. Reduce pressure** (Chapter 6)

Pressure on the stomach can come from outside your body or inside your abdomen but whatever its source, it squashes the stomach and contributes to pushing acid backwards. Abdominal fat is thought to be a significant cause of such pressure. Straining on the toilet or when lifting is another way that pressure can be raised temporarily. There will be some suggestions about how to lift without straining and how to avoid the straining that can be caused by constipation.

**3. Work with gravity** (Chapter 7)

If you're standing or sitting, gravity helps to keep your stomach contents in their proper place but if you bend forward or lie down with a full stomach, you increase the risk of acid back-flow. Most of us could improve the way we reach for things below knee level and the position in which we carry out floor-level tasks. This is looked at in some detail, along with advice about lying down after eating.

**4. Avoid irritants** (Chapter 8)

Whether or not a particular food seems to make reflux worse seems to be highly individual. But if your oesophagus is sore and inflamed, it makes sense to avoid consuming things that are likely to cause further irritation.

**5. Reduce stomach activity** (Chapter 9)

The more your stomach churns, the more likely it is that acid will flow backwards, so there are some suggestions about how to help your stomach rest quietly for more of the time.

**6. Medicines and self-help** (Chapter 10)

There are several medicines that can be bought over the counter and self-medication may have a place in the management of your reflux. There are other medicines that can be prescribed by your doctor. What are these medicines? How do they work? Are these drugs a good option for short-term or long-term control? How, and when, can you use them alongside a self-help campaign?

I suggest you read through these chapters in order and then move on to Chapter 11, which talks about how to approach bringing about the changes that will help you to control your reflux.

# Chapter 5

# Your Diaphragm

I have explained in Chapter 2 how a weak diaphragm can contribute to reflux. In this chapter you will learn how to strengthen and tone your diaphragm so it can play its part in gripping the bottom of your oesophagus and preventing backflow from your stomach.

The role of the diaphragm in helping to prevent reflux has been known for many years but the idea of strengthening it has yet to make its way into mainstream advice. This may be because few researchers have taken an interest. However a study published in 2012 found that a group of reflux patients who practised deep breathing experienced a significant improvement in comfort compared to a control group who did no breathing exercises. Measurements were also taken of the acidity at the bottom of the oesophagus before and after the practice period, and this reduced significantly. This is encouraging, but it would be good to have more research in this area. This chapter will take you beyond simple deep breathing and explain how you can develop a strong, efficient diaphragm.

In a few professions, a powerful diaphragm is essential, opera singing for instance. Free divers too, develop their breathing capacity and train

themselves to stay submerged for several minutes without equipment. These experts demonstrate that it is possible to bring about big improvements.

In very active people, who take regular vigorous exercise that makes them "out of breath", the diaphragm gets some worthwhile exercise. In those who lead more sedentary lives, it rarely works anything near its full capacity, so there's plenty of scope to make it stronger.

As we all know, the only way to make a muscle stronger is to exercise it regularly, starting gradually and building up the work. This chapter takes you through some techniques that exercise the diaphragm. It starts with three fundamental breathing exercises. Then there are some additional things you can do if you'd like some variety.

I suggest that you read the whole chapter before trying out any of the exercises. Then start at the beginning, learning and practising each of the first three exercises in turn. When you feel completely comfortable with each one, you are ready to move on to the next. If you have done something similar before (in yoga, singing or childbirth classes for instance) you will be able to move on quickly. But don't worry if your progress is slow and you're taking a couple of weeks, or more, over each one. Just keep spending a bit of time practising every day and in a few months time your diaphragm will be in much better shape.

The foundation of these exercises is deep, diaphragmatic breathing. This is sometimes known as abdominal breathing because your abdomen moves, passively, in and out when you use your diaphragm. It feels as if your abdomen is filling up with air but the work is done by your diaphragm, not your abdominal muscles.

Muscles adapt to the demands you make on them. If you use them lightly they will lose power and substance. If you use them more they will increase in strength and bulk. Muscles that are well exercised are not only stronger, they also have better "tone". For a demonstration of muscle tone, look at the abdomens of swimmers or boxers. Their abdominal muscles are obviously strong, but they are also "toned", in other words they are tighter than a weak muscle. Even when they are relaxed there is no hint of sagging or paunchiness.

The exercises in this chapter are aimed at developing muscle tone in your diaphragm to strengthen that pinching action at the hiatus. Unlike many exercises, you will not be able to see any physical changes. Instead you should notice an improvement in your reflux symptoms.

Doing the exercises in this chapter just once a week will *not* strengthen and tone your diaphragm and won't help at all with your symptoms. "Little and often" is the only way to proceed if you want to make any muscle stronger.

The good thing is that the basic exercises are not time consuming and can be done almost anywhere, without any special clothing or equipment. Other people won't notice you practising unless they are very observant.

Linking your basic exercises to some regular activity or event will make them part of your daily routine. You could do them while you wait for the lights to change at road junctions, when waiting for food to cook or when advertisements appear on the television.

It's probably better to practise on an empty stomach as your diaphragm can move more freely. Also, if the valve at the entrance to your stomach is very weak or damaged, a strong downward movement of your diaphragm on a full stomach could, in theory, cause reflux. However in most people the inward breath is accompanied by a tightening of the hiatus, which tends to discourage reflux.

When exercising your diaphragm always lie, sit or stand straight (not hunched over or curled into a ball) so you make as much room as possible for it to move.

You might find it helpful to record the instructions and listen while you are learning. Very quickly you will get used to the exercise and won't need to listen to instructions any more.

**The Basic Breath**

If you've studied yoga or singing, or been to childbirth preparation classes, you may have already practised diaphragmatic (or "abdominal") breathing.

The Basic Breath is my shorthand for abdominal/diaphragmatic breathing. It is not difficult to learn and will work your diaphragm to its full capacity.

When you are breathing lightly your diaphragm moves up and down about two or three centimetres. When you do the Basic Breath, it will be moving eight to ten centimetres.

Sit in a comfortable position with your back straight. Alternatively, lie on your back. Place both hands on your abdomen, palms facing inwards with fingers spread out.

Take a deep breath in and feel your abdomen expand beneath your hands. Then let the air flow out smoothly and feel your abdomen moving inwards slightly. If you are wearing tight clothes you may feel your waistband tightening and loosening.

You can breathe in and out through your nose or through your mouth, it doesn't matter. The aim is to get as much movement in your abdomen as possible, without forcing it. You should not be not tensing and relaxing your abdominal muscles – the movement is coming from the piston action of your diaphragm. It's pushing the organs in your abdomen downwards and slightly forwards every time you breathe in.

Now establish a rhythm, breathing in smoothly, expanding your abdomen and then breathing out slowly. Don't force your abdomen in or out and don't sigh when you breathe out.

Imagine your abdominal area becoming barrel-shaped as you breathe in, swelling up in front, around the sides and around the back of your waist.

Try counting as you breathe to help you keep a steady rhythm. Start by counting *in* for four seconds (one and a two and a three and a four) and *out* for four seconds. Take a little pause between breaths and don't rush. Basic Breathing should be done as slowly and smoothly as possible.

Once you are comfortable with this Basic Breathing you can dispense with the hands on your abdomen and, if you wish, the counting.

You can practise in any situation: sitting in a meeting, travelling, watching TV or lying in bed. Frequent practice – little and often - will start to activate and strengthen your diaphragm. Aim to practise for a couple of minutes, several times a day.

**There are a couple of potential problems with learning this type of breathing:**

### 1. Hyperventilation

With any new exercise there is always the possibility of over-doing it and deep breathing is no exception. You're very unlikely to develop sore muscles but you might breathe too quickly and over-breathe or "hyperventilate".

If you take a rapid series of very deep breaths, you alter the delicate balance of oxygen and carbon dioxide in your bloodstream. This imbalance can make you light-headed, dizzy or even cause fainting. This happens because the changes affect the breathing-control centres in your brain, which respond by trying to get you to lie down (and stop being so silly!), hence the faintness.

To avoid hyperventilation, breathe slowly and steadily, with no huffing, no puffing and no sighing. If your breathing is making you feel dizzy, slow it down and breathe out more slowly (count out for 6 instead of 4 for instance).

The important thing is to find a way of breathing deeply *and* slowly that feels relaxed and comfortable for you.

### 2. Trouble getting your abdomen moving

Another problem some people have is that they are in the habit of using their intercostal muscles too much. You will remember that these are the little muscles between your ribs.

Try this: Suck in your abdominal muscles as tightly as you can. Now try to hold them in and take a deep Basic Breath at the same time. Tricky, isn't it, because your tight abdominal muscles are preventing your diaphragm from moving freely. Keeping your abdominals tight, try to breath in and out a few times. You will probably find your body automatically shifts to chest-expanding intercostal breathing because your diaphragm can't move freely. You could get the same effect by wearing a really tight belt or corset.

Natural, relaxed breathing uses the diaphragm. If you then walk up four flights of steps and need to breathe a lot more deeply, your intercostal muscles join in, moving your ribs outwards and helping you to inhale more deeply. They act like a back up when you need extra oxygen. But using them constantly could lead to a weak diaphragm.

If you are not sure about the difference between using your diaphragm and your intercostals, try this:

 Lie on your back in bed or in the bath. Put your hands on your abdomen and do some Basic Breaths. Feel your abdomen moving out and in again with each breath. Carry on with your deep breathing and put both hands on your upper chest with your fingers spread. Notice if there is any movement under your hands. Ideally you should be able to feel little or no movement. Now try to use your intercostal muscles. Breath in sharply each time, as if you were trying to fill your ribcage with air. You should be able to feel a slight expansion under your hands as your ribs lift upwards and slightly outwards. It's only a small movement, a few millimetres, but noticeably different to the lack of movement during abdominal breathing.

You need to avoid this ribcage expansion when doing the work suggested in this chapter. The first step is to recognise it because unless you do, you can't notice yourself doing it and train yourself to avoid it.

Some people tend to use their intercostals a lot. It could be that something like chronic asthma in childhood started them on this path. Or it could be associated with anxiety. Others have trained themselves to hold in their abdominal muscles to look slimmer or because they wear tight clothes that restrict their breathing.

A researcher in the Czech Republic has reported that intercostal breathing tends to open the LOS, which tends to stay closed during diaphragmatic breathing.

If you have identified that you tend to over-use your intercostals, the exercises in this chapter will help you to re-connect with your diaphragm and get it moving again.

And for everyone, always check that you are using your diaphragm and not your intercostals. It will get easier to tell the difference as you gain experience.

Practise the Basic Breath until you are completely confident that you can keep it going comfortably, without using your intercostals, before you move on to the next breathing technique.

**The Extended Breath**

Once you are completely comfortable with the Basic Breath, you are ready to increase the demand on your diaphragm and begin to build up more strength. You are going to do this by taking a deep abdominal breath and then trying to keep breathing in for a few seconds more.

Breathe in deeply until your lungs feel full and your waist area feels barrel-shaped. Keep your throat open and relaxed while you keep trying to breathe in more and more deeply. Push out your abdominal muscles as far as they will go without closing your throat or using your intercostals. Try to squeeze in a bit more air, and a bit more, until it feels as if your abdomen is filled to capacity. Then let the air out (slowly, please).

Always breathe out slowly - no need to huff, puff or sigh. Take a small recovery breath, or two, in between each Extended Breath. Repeat 5-10 times, several times a day.

Try to keep the rest of your body relaxed while you practise. Your shoulders shouldn't move, neither should your upper chest. As you breathe, keep your jaw, hands, arms and shoulders soft and check that you are not frowning or screwing up your face. This is important because it will allow you to practise in public.

The Extended Breath contracts your diaphragm to its limit and then holds it there. It involves a lot more effort than just breathing in deeply and then immediately breathing out. It also requires a lot more work than breathing in and holding your breath in the traditional way, by closing your throat.

Never "hold your breath" by closing off your throat while doing this exercise. When you close your throat you are holding back the air with your throat muscles. Your diaphragm will start to relax, letting your throat muscles do all the work. There is more detail on breath-holding in Chapter 6.

As you get used to doing the Extended Breath, your diaphragm will gradually gain in stamina and your control will improve. You will be able to make the length of your Extended Breath longer as your diaphragm grows stronger.

**Back-to-Front breathing**

Once you are really happy with the Extended Breath, I strongly recommend that you learn this third technique and make it part of your regular, daily practice. I find it easiest to do when lying on my back, so I practise for a few minutes before I get out of bed in the morning.

You might have noticed that I've been using phrases like "imagine the air filling up the back of your waist" and "imagine a barrel shape". I'm going to explain why.

When the diaphragm develops before birth, it forms from three areas of muscle that knit together in the middle to make a single sheet. The central patch is fibrous with three areas of muscle around its sides. There are two big patches at the front and sides that are anchored to the ribs and a smaller patch at the back, known as the crural diaphragm, which is attached to the spine. The oesophagus passes through the crural diaphragm. This is where the hiatus is found and this is the bit that needs to be strengthened in reflux sufferers.

The front patches form the major breathing muscle. The crural diaphragm also moves during breathing, but because it's relatively small, it's not providing much help with breathing. Its importance is that it grips the bottom of your oesophagus at the hiatus.

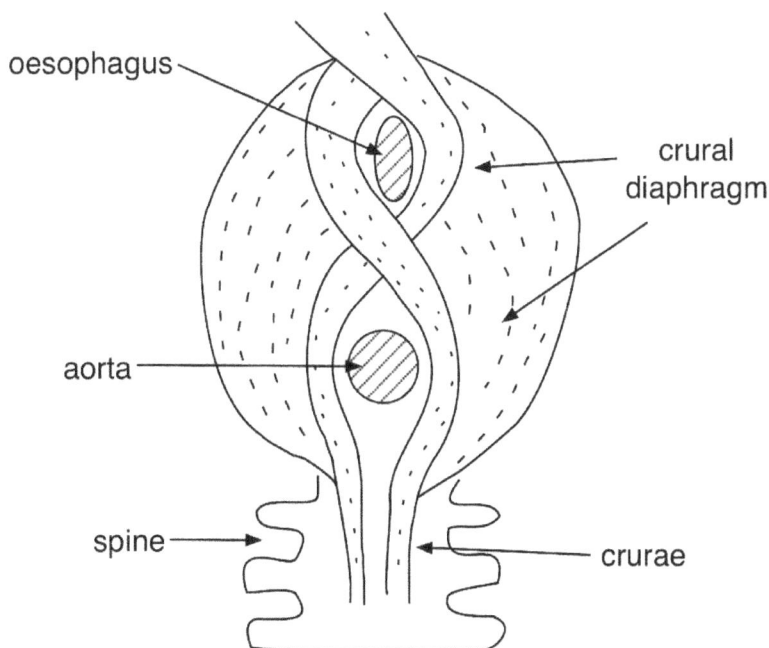

The crural diaphragm includes strips of muscle that curve snugly around your oesophagus and then travel downwards, anchoring firmly into the vertebrae at the back of your waist. These are the crurae, meaning "legs" in Latin, hence the term crural diaphragm. But they are more like crossed fingers, where they wrap around the oesophagus.

The diagram shows the structure of the crural diaphragm as if looking up at it, from below. In it you can see how it includes two fingers of muscle that twine around the oesophagus When learning breathing techniques it often helps to imagine the air moving into different parts of your body. You can use you hands to help the visualisation.

Choose a comfortable position, sitting or lying on your back. Place a hand on your abdomen. Breathe deeply, imagining the air is going into your abdomen, towards your hand. Keep this going, slowly and steadily for about a minute.

Now put a hand on the back of your waist. Breathe in very slowly, towards your hand, imagining the air flowing into that area and then smoothly out again. Your hand may detect a slight movement. Keep the breathing going for a couple of minutes. Now take your hand away and try to get that feeling of breathing into the back of your waist.

When are doing Back-to-Front breathing it feels a little different to the Basic Breath. Your abdomen still expands but it feels as if it's filling up from the back instead of the front.

Here is an alternative visualisation you might like to try:

Close your eyes and, using the Basic Breath, imagine that as you breathe in, the air is filling up the front part of your abdomen. Imagine you can see the air. It's full of sparkles, like a magic spell in a cartoon film. As you breathe in very slowly, picture this sparkly air moving in through your nose, down through your chest, filling up a space in the front part of your abdomen, just beneath the skin. Keep this going for a couple of minutes. Then imagine you have an extra lung at the back of your abdomen. It has a small entrance on the inside of your spine, just above your waistline. Imagine that instead of breathing into the front of your abdomen, you are drawing the sparkly air into your extra lung, until your abdomen feels full. But this time it is filling from the back. Then imagine the sparkly air flowing out again. Keep it going for a couple of minutes.

This kind of breathing is quite tricky to learn so don't get discouraged if it takes you a while to get the knack. It's a bit like learning to wiggle your ears. If you spent a few minutes every day trying to wiggle them, after a few weeks there would be a detectable movement and after a few months of daily practice, ear wiggling would be your party trick. When you start the movement may seem tiny, almost insignificant but if you keep on focussing you will gain control and the movement will seem a lot more obvious.

Make sure you are really familiar with the Basic Breath and have practised the Extended Breath for a while before tacking Back-to-Front Breathing.

As you strengthen your crural diaphragm you may feel those anchoring fingers of muscle tightening against your spine, at the back of your waist. This shows that the area is getting stronger and you are doing the exercise correctly. A fitness instructor would say you have "isolated" the muscle.

If you want to check that the tightening feeling is the right one: your lungs should fill up when you do it. Tightening other core muscles in that waist area won't inflate your lungs, they will tend to have the opposite effect.

Once you have learned Back-to-Front Breathing you can combine it with the Extended Breath technique to get a lot of extra work into the area.

When you have mastered the three techniques, Basic, Extended and Back-to-Front breathing, you need to make them part of your daily life. In this way you will keep your diaphragm in good condition so that does as much as possible to prevent reflux.

Don't worry if it takes you several weeks, or months, to get to this point, just keep practising and there will be a steady improvement in the tone of your diaphragm.

Here are some more things you can try for variety.

**In the tub**

If you have access to a swimming pool, hot tub or bathtub you can use water to help you develop the strength of your diaphragm.

Next time you are in a swimming pool, hang about in the shallow end and try this: Your upper body is vertical and the water comes up to the top of your chest. Practise one of your breathing techniques. You will find that deep breathing is much harder when your trunk is under water because the water pressure is pushing inwards on your chest and abdomen from every direction. This means that your diaphragm has to make a lot more effort to draw air inwards. So this is a good way to build strength.

If you don't have access to a swimming pool or hot tub you can practise in a bathtub. Even if you have water partly covering your abdomen and chest you will get a benefit.

## Go for a walk

Most of the exercises in this book can be done while sitting or standing.

Walking is excellent whole-body exercise and it is easy to incorporate some diaphragm exercises into the rhythm of walking.

While walking, try to co-ordinate your Basic Breath with your stride pattern. For example: breathe in deeply for six strides, and then breathe out, under control, for six strides. Keep it going.

Find a count that suits your body. It may be three strides in and three strides out or you may be counting to eight or nine. This will depend on a lot of factors such as how fast you are walking and your general level of fitness. The rhythm will not be the same as the one that suits you when you're sitting still, as your body is using much more oxygen.

You can adapt this to other kinds of exercise - jogging, cycling, working-out in the gym and so on. Swimming, too, is a very good form of exercise that encourages you to breathe deeply and fully.

## Work against gravity

When you are standing or sitting, gravity helps your diaphragm to work, pulling it downwards. Also, when you are upright, your abdominal organs are in their lowest position, exerting no pressure on your diaphragm.

If you lie flat, the assistance from gravity disappears and some of the weight of your abdominal organs shifts onto your diaphragm. So if you practise when you are lying flat your diaphragm has to work a bit harder and there is an extra benefit.

**Bridge**

If your symptoms are under control, this advanced exercise will build strength and stamina in your diaphragm and help to keep your symptoms at bay.

The bridge exercise will tip up your body so your diaphragm has to work even harder against gravity. It will inevitably tilt your stomach above the hiatus and could encourage back-flow of acid. So use your judgement to decide whether you are ready to try it. If you are experiencing a lot of acid reflux, my advice is to wait until you have got it under control.

If you do decide to have a go, I would recommend you do it with a completely empty stomach, first thing in the morning.

Do not do this is you have very high blood pressure or if you have ever suffered from a stroke as it could increase pressure in the blood vessles in your head.

You will need to be on a firm surface, a floor or a mat, not a bed or sofa. Your feet need to grip, so either work with bare feet or wear soft shoes with ridged soles.

This is one of the most simple and useful yoga poses. It has several benefits, beyond working your diaphragm. It strengthens your lower back, buttocks and thighs and encourages flexibility in your spine. So, as an exercise, it's good value.

Lie on your back on the floor with your arms by your sides, your knees bent and your feet planted firmly on a non-slip surface. Remove any pillows or other padding from under your head. Move your feet and knees apart so there is a small space between them (same amount of space between your knees as there is between your feet). Now move your arms a small distance away from your hips, and place your palms on the mat beside you. Lift your head a little and push your chin down towards your chest, so that you don't squash the back of your neck. Place your head back down but keep looking in the general direction of your feet. Now you are ready to begin making a bridge.

Flatten the back of your waist into the floor. It should be firmly against the floor, with no gaps if possible. Tighten your buttocks and push with your feet so your hips lift off the floor. Keep pushing up, trying to lift your hips off the floor as you move your body up towards a 45 degree angle. Use your arms and hands to brace yourself if necessary. Your chin stays tucked towards your chest and your head does not move.

Once you have lifted your hips, keep tightening your buttocks and try to hold your best position for a count of four before lowering, slowly, back to the floor. As you go down, imagine you are curling down, one vertebra at a time, with your buttocks touching last, before you relax.

As you practise this exercise, breathe in slowly and deeply as you lift up. Breathe out, under control, as you go down.

If you can't make a 45 degree slope, find an angle that suits you - the important thing is that you should be able to hold still and steady while you work your diaphragm. It may take time to build up the strength to hold this position.

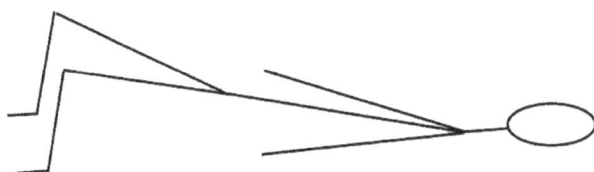

When you have practised this sequence of movements and you feel steady in your final position, you can start to hold the position and do one of the three fundamental breathing techniques. Regular practice will make it easier.

You will feel your diaphragm exercising harder, working against gravity and pushing your abdominal organs uphill. There is significantly more effort involved than when you are breathing in an upright position and this extra effort will make the muscle stronger.

It's interesting to notice something else in this position. When upright, if you try to fully empty your lungs you have to squeeze in with your abdominal muscles to press out the last bit of air. In the full bridge position you don't have to do this. As you breathe out, the weight of your abdominal organs rests on your diaphragm and fully empties your lungs.

I'll emphasis again that this last exercise is suitable for people who are fairly physically active and who have got symptoms pretty much under control. If you have a bad hernia or uncontrolled acid reflux, you may want to give it a miss.

Students of yoga (or just idle observers) will know that there are several other inverted yoga postures that are more extreme than bridge. Examples are headstands and shoulder stands. I do not recommend either of these unless you are under the personal instruction of an experienced yoga teacher.

**Summary of chapter:**

Strengthen your diaphragm by learning the three breathing exercises and practising for short periods several times a day.

# Chapter 6

# Reduce Pressure

Any extra pressure on your stomach will tend to increase the tendency for acid to flow backwards. If you've ever come across a practical joke known as a "whoopee cushion" you will be able to picture how this happens. A whoopee cushion is a flat rubber balloon with a flat tube to allow for the passage of air (if you haven't seen one, look it up on the Internet – or better still buy one and enjoy the fun). Once you have blown into it, the tube remains closed without needing to be tied because the gentle elasticity of the rubber keeps it flat. Then you pop it under your victim's seat cushion. When they sit down, pressure on the cushion increases and the air is forced out of the tube creating a loud, flatulent sound.

It's a similar mechanism at the LOS. Under normal conditions the end of the oesophagus is collapsed. It's kept closed by gentle squeezing of the diaphragm and the rubbery walls at the bottom of the oesophagus. But this combination only acts as a weak valve. A little bit of extra pressure on the stomach can cause its contents to escape and they more likely to escape upwards because the pyloric valve, at the other end of the stomach, is much stronger.

Your stomach lies next to the largest and most solid abdominal organ, the liver, and both stomach and liver are tucked under your even-firmer ribs. Below these, your other abdominal organs are packed in neatly, with the whole lot held in place by the muscles of your back and abdomen. So although the stomach is an elastic bag, pressure on it can easily affect the naturally weak LOS.

Extra pressure can come from outside of the abdomen or from the inside. There are a number of things that you can do to minimise pressure and so help reduce the amount of reflux you are suffering. Some of them are easy to accomplish while others require determination.

### Don't over-eat

The most obvious one is not to over-fill your stomach. An unusually large meal takes up a lot of space and over-stretches your stomach. This will increase the pressure exerted by your stomach walls and put pressure on your LOS. So stick to normal-sized meals and don't indulge in eating contests.

### Avoid tight clothes

Another easy one is to avoid squashing your abdomen with clothing. If you want keep your symptoms to a minimum, resist the temptation to wear anything that presses on your abdomen or waist.

### Avoid:

- tight waistbands

- tight belts

- tight jeans or skirts

- corsets

- elasticated foundation garments ("magic knickers", "shapewear" etc)

Your waistline will be at its slimmest in the morning when yesterday's meals have been digested and you're a little dehydrated. As the day goes on and you've consumed various meals and drinks, your clothes may feel tighter. So when you dress in the morning allow for this or "slip into something more comfortable" later in the day. If you'll be sitting all day, make allowances for this too, as clothes that are a perfect fit when you get dressed inevitably feel a bit tighter when you sit down.

**Lose weight**

Now something that is rather more challenging: losing weight.

When you gain weight, fat cells in different parts of the body are involved. Sometimes the cells are just under the skin, forming subcutaneous fat. It's the kind you can pinch, particularly on the abdomen, where it can form rolls.

If you have this kind of fat around your waist it may make your symptoms worse because every time you bend forward it will squash your stomach. You might even feel, when sitting, that there is a cushion of fat pushing inwards at your waistline. This kind of fat can also prompt people to feel that they should wear tight garments to make them look slimmer.

Another kind of fat can develop *inside* the abdominal cavity, wrapped around the internal organs. It lies underneath your abdominal muscles and you can't pinch it. If you have a lot of this internal fat, you'll be developing a paunch that sticks out in front like a pregnancy and presses on your stomach from below. This is sometimes referred to as a "beer belly" but it is not caused by beer consumption (although beer contains a lot of calories so it can contribute to weight gain.)

If your abdomen bulges upwards when you are lying flat on your back, it's a sign that you have internal fat. Some overweight people have both types of fat.

Internal fat is very bad for reflux because it occupies space inside your abdominal cavity and crowds your stomach. The pressure it causes could also contribute to the formation of a hiatus hernia or make an existing hernia worse.

Men are more likely than women to develop abdominal fat and they are also more likely to develop cancer of the oesophagus (see Chapter 3). We don't know for sure that the belly fat is the main cause but the suspicion is fairly strong.

Being seriously overweight is linked to increased tendency to reflux but even a little bit of excess weight might be unhelpful.

There is some research evidence about the benefits of losing weight. For instance a very big, long-term study of the health of American nurses found that, in women whose weight was in the normal range:

- An increase in weight of 10-15 pounds led to a 40% increase in reflux symptoms.

- A decrease in weight of 10-15 pounds led to a 40% decrease in reflux symptoms.

- Women in the study who were overweight were 2-3 times more likely to suffer from reflux than those of normal weight.

The message is clear: if you have a tendency to reflux, gaining weight will probably make it worse and losing some weight is one of the best ways to improve things.

Excess fat is linked statistically to a range of unpleasant "diseases of civilisation" and reflux is one more to add to the list. Maybe the regular discomfort of reflux will be prompt you to tackle it and at the same time reduce your risk of developing Type 2 diabetes and coronary artery disease.

Losing weight requires determination but there is plenty of advice available on how to do it. Crash diets, leading to sudden weight loss, are known to be poor long-term solutions, with weight tending to creep back on. Many people find it helpful to join a programme where they are supported to eat more healthily and to take more exercise. If you feel your eating is difficult to control it may be worth looking at some kind of counselling to help you understand the reasons you overeat and to support your efforts to change.

**Adapt your exercise routine**

Exercise is good for you in many ways and *moderate* exercise seems to have a protective effect against reflux. Nobody knows why but it could be the result of exercising the diaphragm during physical activity. Swimming and brisk walking are both great ways to take moderate exercise.

Vigorous exercise, though, has a tendency to increase reflux symptoms. This could be due to changes in body chemistry; changes in the activity of the stomach or the effect of bouncing up and down. You can imagine stomach contents would slosh around when someone is jogging and indeed one study found that runners are more likely to suffer reflux than cyclists.

Any exercise that squeezes in your abdominal muscles has the potential to squash your stomach, cause reflux and put pressure on a hernia.

If you want do sit-ups ("crunches") the best time is first thing in the morning, on a completely empty stomach. If fact, it's a good idea to have an empty stomach when you do any vigorous exercise. If you are concerned about the appearance of your slightly rounded stomach, it's better to tone your muscles and improve your posture, rather than relying on foundation garments.

Lying on your front in an exercise class could also put pressure on your stomach, depending on the amount of fat you have in that area. If you are not comfortable lying face down, don't do that part of the class.

Forward bends in classes may not help. Consider whether you really want to bend forward from the waist from a standing position, squashing your stomach and tilting it above your oesophagus. If you are bending forward from a sitting position in yoga class, keep your head raised and keep looking forward, rather than trying to get your head down to your knees. The movement should come from your hips, not your spine.

The "pose of a child" in yoga, in which you are curled up in a ball, facing the mat, will put a lot of pressure on your stomach unless you are very slim *and* have an empty stomach. I recommend that, if you really want to do this, or any other forward bending, you should only do so on an empty stomach.

**Improve your posture**

Poor posture puts pressure on your stomach because when you slouch forwards, your ribs and some of the weight of your upper body inevitably rest on your stomach and squash it. If you spend a lot of your day sitting with poor posture, this could be contributing to your reflux.

Try this: Sit up, with a very straight back, near the edge of a dining chair. Place your left hand on your lower left ribs. This is where your stomach and the bottom of your oesophagus are positioned.

Now, keeping your hand there, relax forward into a full slouch, with your spine curved and the weight of your upper body resting on the back part of your buttocks. Notice how far the front of your rib cage drops down. Imagine how your ribs are pressing onto your stomach. Now slowly sit up straight and picture how your rib cage is lifting off your stomach, giving it a lot more space.

Sitting up straight may make the muscles in your upper back feel tired. This is a sign that you haven't been using them to support your upper body. It's also an indication that there's a lot you could do to improve your posture.

Good posture is not common in Western cultures. Dancers, singers, musicians and athletes stand out as exceptions amongst adults. Most of us sit too much and, when in a sitting position, rely on chairs to support our backs, rather than using our postural muscles. Look at a group of people who are sitting on benches (bleachers) or on the ground. How many straight spines can you see? You'll probably observe that most adults will be slouching. In the section below I am concentrating on improving sitting posture because you are more likely to slouch when sitting than standing.

To improve your posture you need to sit *as though* you have great posture. Do this often enough and your postural muscles will become stronger and you will start to hold that straight-backed position naturally.

Good sitting posture starts, literally, at the bottom. If you are sitting in a slumped position, you are probably resting your weight not on your sitting bones, but on the flesh of your upper buttocks. By tilting off this area and onto your sitting bones, you immediately improve your posture. Here's how to do it:

Sit up straight on a dining chair with a big gap between your spine and the back of the chair. Place both feet on the ground. You should be balanced on your sitting bones, two bumps at the bottom of your pelvis. They are found in the middle of your buttocks. Rock a little on the chair and try to locate them. If you can't feel them, try sitting on your fingers. The sitting bones are the smooth, rounded, hard bumps.

Once you are balanced on your sitting bones you can think about your upper body.

Now try this:

Rest your hands in a relaxed position in your lap or on the arms of your chair.

With your weight resting on your sitting bones straighten your back. Notice how the muscles in your back have to work to keep you upright. Relax your shoulders, let them roll backwards and down (just a centimetre or two) and lift your chest a centimetre or two (lift it, don't stick it out). Remind yourself how lifting your rib cage makes even more space for your stomach. Now maintain this upright sitting until your back muscles start to ache. This may be quite a brief period. Relax, take a short rest and then repeat.

The simplest way to strengthen your back and improve your posture is to do this simple practice as often as possible. Find times to fit it into your every day life - when you are sitting in the car, at your desk, in meetings, at meal times or in front of the TV or computer. Don't let the chair do the sitting for you. If you can get into the habit of sitting like this several times a day, every day, you'll feel a rapid improvement in the strength and stamina of your back muscles and good sitting posture will become a habit.

I've been working on this for a couple of years now. When sitting in the car, or at a dining table, I take this upright position without having to remind myself. But I still have to correct my posture from time to time when sitting at my desk.

Some people have additional challenges. Some women carry additional weight around the bust. If this is your issue, make sure you are wearing a good bra, to help distribute the weight as best you can.

People with a lot of abdominal fat (or those in advanced pregnancy) may have slightly distorted posture in which their back is more arched than it should be and the abdominal wall is over stretched. The remedy for this is weight loss (or giving birth) and then working to strengthen the postural and core muscles.

You may find that your seating is not helping. If you are doing a lot of sitting on soft furniture, or a car seat that is a bit bucket-shaped it may encourage you sit in a way that squashes your stomach. Think about how you can use cushions to get yourself into more of a right-angle while you work on your ability to sit in a more active way.

**Avoid constipation and straining**

Pressure can result from straining when you have a bowel movement. It's natural to hold your breath when you do this. This breath holding increases pressure inside your abdomen and helps to expel faeces. But most of the work is done by the peristaltic action of your lower bowel. If breath holding is prolonged or amounts to "straining" it is bad for reflux and for any kind of hernia.

I have sometimes seen this advice to reflux sufferers:

"In order to strengthen your diaphragm, you should practise blowing up party balloons. Or pretend to do this, without the balloons."

The only bit about this that could help is the part where you breathe in deeply. Blowing into a balloon (particularly if it is a real balloon) will put a lot of pressure on your stomach and is likely to do much more harm than good.

This is what happens when you blow up a balloon:

As you breathe in, your diaphragm moves down, flattens and tightens around your lower oesophagus. Then, when you start to blow into the balloon, your diaphragm will relax and rise up (pushing the air gently out of your lungs). At the same time you are tightening bands of abdominal muscle. These push inwards and upwards, as if you were being laced into a tight corset. This exerts an upward force on stomach, diaphragm and lungs. If the balloon is a real one, you are working against the resistance of its rubber walls, so your abdominal muscles push harder and harder. If your LOS mechanism is not in good shape it's quite possible that this activity could cause reflux. Your diaphragm cannot "blow up balloons" because it can only contract downwards. It has no ability to push upwards, or breathe out with force All it can do is relax into its highest position. It's those abdominal muscles that are doing the blowing-up. So if someone asks you to blow up real balloons for their party, pass the job on to someone else.

Blowing up balloons is one small step away from "straining".

When you "strain", you breathe in and then close the muscles in your larynx to block the escape of air. You then push inwards and upwards with those bands of abdominal muscle. It's like trying to blow up a particularly tough balloon that just won't co-operate, but instead of forcing the air into a balloon you're blocking its escape from your lungs. This builds very high pressure in your abdomen and chest. As it builds, you go red in the face and veins start to bulge in your neck and face. You can see this happening in Olympic weightlifters as they strive towards the limit of their strength. The medical term for straining is the Valsalva Manoeuvre.

Straining has dramatic effects throughout your body. The high pressure in your abdomen and chest disrupts the flow of blood back to the heart. Hence the red face and bulging veins. The blood is literally backing up in your veins and your blood pressure shoots up. During the second stage of labour, mothers strain or "push" (it's also sometimes called "bearing down") to help the baby into the world. They sometimes strain so hard that they burst little blood vessels in the whites of their eyes.

When you are mid-strain the pressure will be equal in your chest and abdomen. But the force that creates that pressure is applied upwards from your abdominal muscles and will inevitably squeeze your stomach. Imagine a balloon, half filled with water, with a clothes peg or hairgrip closing its neck. If the balloon is gripped hard enough, the air and water will be pushed out. I therefore recommend that you avoid straining.

So after that digression, let's return to the bathroom.

Your lower bowel has a mind of its own. I mean this quite literally. The gut wall contains a neural network, of huge complexity, that operates fairly independently from the rest of the nervous system. Its job is to sense what is happening at various stages of digestion and to control digestion and peristalsis. It's like a computer controlling an automated chemical factory. When the bowel is getting full, it sends faeces down into your rectum. This sends a message to your conscious brain that it's time to find a suitable place and position. When the moment is right, the sphincters that control the anus are released and strong peristaltic contractions of the bowel push out the faeces. A little bit of extra straining pressure may help, but it doesn't supply the main force. The peristaltic action of the bowel does most of the work.

The action of your lower bowel works best when the faeces are bulky and fairly soft giving its muscles something to push against. It also works best when you feel relaxed and safe because the central nervous system can interfere with the smooth operation of the nervous system in the bowel.

Any degree of constipation (hard, dry or small faeces, or a sluggish bowel) is going to encourage you to strain. This is not going to help your reflux symptoms, nor will it help a hernia, if you have one.

The first line of attack on constipation is to eat a high-fibre diet. This will produce larger, softer faeces that will stimulate your bowel and help it to work more efficiently. Various studies have shown that that people who eat more fibre tend to get less reflux. As with most of these studies we can't be sure that the high-fibre diet is the *cause* of less reflux. But the connection between fibre and reflux could be that constipated people strain and that straining increases the incidence of reflux. One of the ways doctors diagnose oesophagitis pain is to ask "does it get worse if you strain, lift or bend?"

**What is dietary fibre?**

Fibre is a term used for something that is present in food but cannot be digested by humans. Although it doesn't nourish us, it helps the bowel to function in a healthy way. Foods that contain little or no fibre include peeled potatoes, white rice, meat, fish, eggs, cheese, fats, oils and things made of white flour. So if these are the things that make up your current diet, you may well be constipated.

Nutrition experts tell us that are two kinds of fibre: insoluble and soluble. But it may be useful to think of *three* different categories: roughage, cellulose and "soluble fibre". Both roughage and cellulose are referred to as "insoluble fibre" but they are quite different substances. What they have in common is that they absorb water, bulk up faeces and prevent constipation.

## 1. Roughage

This is fibrous, indigestible vegetable matter such as bran. It absorbs water, bulks up and softens faeces and so stimulates the healthy action of the bowel. It includes husks, woody bits, peel, pith and vegetable skins. It can be obtained from whole grains (brown bread, pasta and rice), whole seeds, beans, bran, nuts, fruits and vegetables with skins and seeds. Some people find this kind of fibre a bit irritating to the bowel (for instance if they suffer from irritable bowel syndrome) but for most people it's a normal, healthy part of the diet.

## 2. Cellulose

This is the stuff that makes up the walls of all plant cells. It's a kind of carbohydrate that is indigestible by humans.

If you have ever mixed a bucket of wallpaper paste you have come across dried cellulose because that is exactly what wallpaper paste is made of. You will have noticed how a dry, granular cellulose soaks up a surprisingly large quantity of water and makes a bucketful of paste. It's a gelatinous, gloopy substance, without a single fibre in sight. Gel-like drinks designed to alleviate constipation consist mainly of cellulose.

It's fairly easy to imagine that cellulose behaves in the bowel,,retaining water and helping to bulk up and soften faeces. In this way it gently helps the lower bowel to function happily.

If you consume cellulose gel drinks you do need to drink significantly more fluid than you would otherwise do (remember, it's absorbent, like wallpaper paste). If you are increasing the amount of fibre-rich food in your diet, increase your fluid intake a little but there is no need to drink excessively. The extra fluid does not have to be water. If tea were not a good way to re-hydrate the body, many of us would have gone to an early grave.

Active adults often seem to worry about water consumption and walk around clutching water bottles, but there is no scientific or medical reason for consuming extra water unless you are taking vigorous and prolonged exercise (like running a marathon). You just need to replace the amount you lose in 24 hours via sweating, breathing, faeces and urine. Producing additional amounts of dilute urine has no added benefits. An average woman needs about a litre and a half of fluid a day including the water in food. When people talk about "eight glasses a day" they are not talking about large glasses, they are talking about small wine glasses or teacups (200ml).

Those most likely to drink too little seem to me to be older people who have mobility problems. They may restrict their intake because getting out of their chair is painful and they want to limit their trips to the toilet, or it's difficult to walk to the kitchen and make a drink. Others are dependent on other people to provide them with drinks, and may not want to ask.

The thing to remember about water if you are a reflux sufferer, is that a few mouthfuls of plain water can wash acid out of your oesophagus and get rid of a burning sensation or other reflux- related pain. So it can act as an instant remedy.

It's best to get the fibre you need by eating a balanced diet. Whole fruits and vegetables provide vitamins and minerals that are lacking in gel drinks or tablespoons of bran.

If you have a sensitive bowel and want to avoid roughage, you should go for cellulose-rich, high-fibre foods that are low in roughage such as:

- Tender, leafy foods such as lettuce, bean sprouts, cabbage and spinach

- Peeled and seeded tomatoes and cucumbers

- Stoned and peeled fruit such as apples, pears, plums and peaches

- Melon, marrow and the pumpkin family

- Citrus fruit with pith removed

- Soups and smoothies made without seeds, skin, pips

- Onions

- Mushrooms

### 3. Soluble fibre

This term refers to a range of plant-based substances, which can't be digested by humans but can be broken down by "friendly" bacteria in your bowel. The bacteria produce short-chain fatty acids, vitamins and other substances that are beneficial to our health. "Soluble" is not a very precise word but it's the one in current use. It's found in things like oats, beans, lentils, peas, hummus, dhal and nuts. These all contain the other kinds of fibre as well.

Because this kind of fibre feeds friendly bacteria it also stimulates them to produce gas. Baked beans are famous for having this effect. Intestinal gas is normal and an increase can be a side effect of increasing your fibre intake. Don't make too many changes to your diet at once because you might find the effects a bit sudden. Adjust the type and quantity of high-fibre foods until your bowels are working well, but not *too* well.

**How much fibre do you need to prevent constipation?**

The daily recommended fibre intake for adults is, in the UK, *at least* 18 grams. But if you look at the recommendations of government advisory bodies around the world you see figures as high as 38 grams a day (in Australia, for adult men). In fact, nobody knows the ideal amount needed to maintain bowel health and it may vary between individuals. My grandchildren both eat the same diet but one tends to be constipated while the other has never had the problem.

The best way to meet the recommended levels is to eat a combination of vegetables, fruit, seeds, beans and whole grains.

Most of us also eat some processed food products and some of these claim to add fibre to your diet. There are strict European rules about how these foods are described:

*A claim that a food is a "source of fibre"*, or any claim likely to have the same meaning for the consumer, may only be made where the product contains at least 3 grams of fibre per 100 grams. ?

*A claim that a food is "high in fibre"*, or any claim likely to have the same meaning for the consumer, may only be made where the product contains at least 6 grams of fibre per 100 grams.

In other words if you eat a bowl of "high fibre" cereal containing 100 grams of cereal, you only get 6 grams of fibre.

Just to add to the confusion, the word "multigrain" appears on some cereals but does not mean "high in fibre". It just means they are made from a variety of cereal sources (which could be low-fibre wheat flour, rice flour, corn flour and so on). It's an example of clever marketing.

When buying processed foods, the fibre per serving will probably be shown (in tiny writing) on the label. Then *all* you have to do is work out whether your serving size is the same as their serving size (by using a scales and weighing your portion), and do any calculations to adjust – a minor mathematical challenge. It's even more tricky with non-processed foods that don't have labels. So the best method, in my view, is not to count grams but to increase your dietary fibre until your constipation is cured.

**What does a high fibre diet look like?**

This would be typical for me:

- Breakfast – porridge with sultanas
- Lunch – sandwich (maybe with a tomato) or, for a big fibre-boost, beans on toast
- Evening meal – burger with a big helping of home-made salad, made from grated cabbage with added walnuts and raisins. Followed by some fruit.

**Psychology and constipation**

If a high-fibre diet doesn't cure your constipation it's possible that psychological factors may be the cause. Stress and relaxation influence the action of the bowel and so does your body clock. As well as having "a mind of its own", your bowel is linked to your brain. So it's no surprise that its workings are complex and sensitive.

Psychological causes of constipation include:

## 1. Anxiety and stress

It's well known that extreme fear can cause "intestinal hurry" but lower levels of tension can have the opposite effect. If you don't feel relaxed and safe, your bowel may refuse to perform. The tension of having to rush to leave the house in the morning could cause problems for some people. An unfamiliar environment, or using a toilet that's not very private can bring normal bowel action to a complete halt, sometimes for days. On-going anxiety about something that has nothing at all to do with toilets (am I going to fail my exams?) can also slow bowel action. So sitting on the toilet, worrying about whether or not you're bowel is going to work properly, is likely to be counter-productive.

Getting up a bit earlier in the morning could give you time to relax in the bathroom. Some people sit on the toilet and read a magazine or do a puzzle to help them stay relaxed. This is very useful as it occupies the conscious mind and lets the rest of your nervous system get on with emptying your bowel, without interference.

## 2. Lack of a habit

A healthy bowel usually has a fairly regular pattern or "bowel habit" that is driven by a number of factors including the body clock. If you have ever been on a long trip by plane you may have noticed that your bowel takes a few days to catch up. It suffers from jet lag and doesn't work normally until your body clock has started to adjust to the new time zone. Some night-shift workers also complain of a disrupted bowel habit. An irregular lifestyle without a regular morning routine could also disrupt the process.

Eating breakfast can help to stimulate the whole digestive system into action. So if you rush out in the morning without eating, this may be another unhelpful factor.

The other part of "bowel habit" seems to be a conditioned response. You probably remember hearing about Pavlov and his dogs. He paired dinner with a bell and after a while the dogs salivated whenever they heard the bell. The interesting thing about this was that salivation is involuntary. They were not learning a trick to get a reward. The same kind of conditioning can happen in humans. There are probably millions of people whose bowels are conditioned to start working at the sound of the alarm clock or the taste of their first coffee or cigarette of the day. Opening the newspaper to the crossword page seems to work for some. For others there may be a conditioned response triggered by going into their own bathroom and sitting on their own toilet. Then they go on holidays, the routine is different and the bathroom is different and the conditioned response just doesn't kick in.

Having a morning routine may help to establish a conditioned response.

You could try getting up at the same time and eating and drinking the same things in the morning and see if your bowel responds. If your routine includes your book of puzzles, take it with you when you travel.

### 3. Ignoring the urge

It's also possible to train yourself to be constipated. This can happen if you repeatedly ignore the urge to empty your bowel. Everyone probably does this now and again but if it's a regular occurrence you can train your brain to ignore the feeling of needing to go. Imagine someone who didn't allow enough time in the morning. They are running late so instead of sitting on the toilet and relaxing for five minutes, they rush out of the house. Then they get the urge to go when they are half way to work, which is highly inconvenient. When they get to work they don't really want to retreat to the staff toilets as soon as they arrive. So the urge is suppressed and it soon passes so the bowel remains un-emptied for another day. If they do this several days in succession and the brain may start to ignore those "its time to go" messages and chronic constipation can set in.

In a few people there are complicating medical factors that make it difficult to overcome constipation difficult. Examples are diseases that slow the bowel and drugs (such as codeine) that reduce bowel activity. But in otherwise healthy people, constipation can usually be tackled by the simple measures that I have described. So, to recap, this is how to encourage your bowel to work naturally so that you are not tempted to strain on the toilet:

- Eat a high fibre diet

- Establish a regular morning routine

- Allow yourself a period of peace and privacy in the bathroom

- Do a puzzle, or read a magazine (the same thing every day)

- Try not to ignore the urge to go

**Summary of chapter:**

DO

- Lose some weight so that you are not carrying excess fat around your waist

- Learn to sit with good posture

- Deal with any constipation

DON'T

- Over fill your stomach

- Wear tight clothing

- Gain weight

- Strain when using the toilet

# Chapter 7

# Work With Gravity

We live our lives under the influence of gravity. It's a very strong force, like a powerful magnet, pulling downwards on our bodies from the moment we are born.

When you're in an upright position, gravity helps to keep your stomach contents in place. It's easy to imagine though, that if your LOS is weak and you lie down, bend forward or stand on your head, liquid in your stomach could flow backwards.

In this chapter we look at ways in which you can work with gravity to minimise your symptoms.

**Improve the way you bend and lift**

You may have noticed that reflux-related discomfort or pain is often increased by bending forward at the waist. One of the questions that doctors use to aid diagnosis of reflux-related pain is: "Does the pain get worse when you bend forward?"

You may have noticed that when you bend forward, particularly over a full stomach, you experience a gush of reflux in your throat. Bending from the waist squashes your abdomen. It's a double hit. You're increasing the pressure on your stomach at the same time as reducing the anti-reflux effect of an upright position. Doing it on a full stomach is even worse. If you are bending like this many times a day, it may well be contributing to giving you a sore oesophagus by the evening.

One morning I started counting the number of times I needed to reach something at floor level:

- Getting oats out of the cupboard and replacing them - 2

- Getting milk in and out of fridge - 4

- Emptying the dishwasher - 6

- Picking up clothes I dropped last night - 3

- Picking up shampoo bottle and replacing it on floor of shower - 2

- Getting dressed - 6

- Plugging in hairdryer - 1

- Picking up bag - 1

It's very easy to do 20-30 bending movements before the working day begins, which may not get your reflux self-help off to a great start.

However we all need to do tasks like tying shoelaces; retrieving items from low shelves; picking things up off the floor; attending to children or doing the gardening. So how can you accomplish these tasks without bending from the waist?

One thing you can do is just stop and think. In other words, train yourself to become more aware. Instead of bending from the waist to untie your trainers, sit down, keep your back straight and lift up your foot. Stop dropping clothes on the floor and start putting them in the laundry basket or on a hanger. If there are things you use every day that are kept on your lowest shelves, could you re-organise your storage? It might make more sense for you to stretch up rather than bend down.

But making creative adaptations is not going to cover all situations.

If you want to reduce the contribution that bending is making to your reflux, you need to find ways to bend that keep your upper body upright.

One option, if you are in good physical shape, is squatting.

If you watch a toddler playing, you will notice that they will often squat rather than bend. Squatting is a natural movement for humans and it's normal in both adults and children in poorer countries. For them it's easy. They work in this position and may squat to eat their meals or chat with their neighbours. They probably use squatting toilets rather than pedestals. Their joints flex easily and their leg muscles are strong because they have been squatting all their lives. Those of us who grow up with chairs and pedestal toilets tend to lose the strength and flexibility needed to squat.

Squatting is only a good idea if you can do so safely, without losing your balance or hurting your knees. If you have vulnerable knee joints, it's best avoided. Always squat with your feet well apart, to give more stability. If you have fat around your waist, don't squat in a way that puts more pressure on it.

I strongly recommend that if you want to practise squatting, you do so with a hand on a table, sink or work surface to help you to balance.

Put one hand on a solid object for support, place your feet and your knees wide apart, keep your back straight and bend your knees. Keep your knees wide apart as you sink down – but only go down to your comfortable limit. Go up onto your toes if you need to. When you are ready to come up, push smoothly up again, keeping your back upright.

You legs may feel weak. If so, this is a great way to gradually strengthen them.

However re-learning to squat is probably beyond the capacity of many people. Kneeling is an easier option for getting down to ground level.

Full kneeling is a useful position if you have to stay at floor level for a while - to clean up a mess, play with a child or weed the garden. Some gardeners use kneeling pads. If you are doing a prolonged task, take frequent breaks to rest your knees.

For a quicker bend you may like to try the half-kneel. The aim is to have one knee on the ground and the other leg bent at a right angle, with the foot flat on the floor. This can work well for tasks like picking up a sock or emptying the dishwasher.

Here's how to get in and out of the half-kneel. Take a step back, tuck your back toes under and sink down, gracefully, onto you back knee, keeping your spine straight. Your front leg will bend into a right angle. Do your small task and then push with your toes and with both legs as you rise up smoothly. You can push with your hand on the forward knee, or on any stable nearby object.

This movement may take a little practice but it doesn't require great flexibility or athletic ability. If you do it regularly, your leg muscles will get stronger and the movement will get easier. Part of the challenge is the mental one. You have to become much more aware and remind yourself to move differently.

Again I recommend that you always practise this with your hand on a solid object until you are confident that you have the strength and control needed.

If you have physical limitations that mean neither squatting nor kneeling is possible, I suggest you use a low stool to perch on. Place it in front of the low level task. Lower yourself into a sitting position and then do the task. Or get a grabber device to use when picking up items from the floor.

A final word – if you know that you are planning to do a lot of gardening or taking care of a two-year-old, avoid over-filling your stomach.

**How can you lift without straining?**

Sometimes you need to bend down to pick up a heavier item - a child, a bag of shopping or a sack of compost.

When lifting heavy items, people often hold their breath, or grunt – in other words they strain (see Chapter 6). This obviously contributes to the risk of reflux. In a study of people doing a great deal of sport, weight lifters experienced more reflux than runners or cyclists.

Think of ways to *avoid* lifting such as:

- Asking someone else to do the lifting, or to help you.

- Slide a heavy object instead of lifting it. (put your back against it and use your legs to push it maybe?)

- Encouraging a child to walk instead of being picked up and carried.

- If a child falls over, squat, kneel or sit on the floor to comfort them but don't lift them.

- Don't overload shopping bags – break up the load into more bags

If you *must* lift, then learn to do it in a way that avoids the evil combination of full stomach *plus* bending forward *plus* breath-holding.

If your job involves lifting, your employer should provide you with training to ensure you know how to lift safely.

The general aim is to lift with a straight back using the muscles below your waist to do the work, and keep breathing. Get as close to the object as possible, bend your knees and keep your back straight throughout. Do your lifting slowly without any sudden jerking movements.

Your brain will probably want you to take the easy option – bending from the waist and using your back muscles. The only answer is to lift consciously and deliberately, thinking about the way you are using your body and thinking about the fact you want to avoid reflux. Do this often enough and a new habit will establish itself.

**Bed-time woes**

Some reflux sufferers find their symptoms are worse at night. It could be that they are suffering from the cumulative effect of the day's episodes of reflux and heartburn sets in late in the day. An obvious backflow of acid when you are lying down is a sign that the protective mechanisms in your oesophagus are in poor shape and you may need to talk to a surgeon.

Once your stomach has finished processing the last meal of the day it will go into a prolonged rest period - shrunk down to sock size, relaxing its muscles and containing very little gastric juice. So try to have your last meal of the day at least three hours before bed-time, preferably four hours, and avoid evening snacks and drinks. This will give your stomach a chance to empty itself completely and settle down for the night before you lie down in bed. Think, too, about the size of your evening meal. Does it make sense to have your biggest meal at this time?

I realise it might be difficult to give up snacks during the evening. TV adverts for chocolate don't help and neither does evening socialising. But if you are having uncomfortable nights, you have a strong incentive to break the evening-snacking habit.

Another common bit of advice that is commonly given to night-time reflux sufferers is to raise the head of your bed to get a bit of help from gravity. There is some evidence that this is useful if you suffer at night.

You may have to use a bit of creativity to raise the head end of your bed (planks? bricks?). There is also the possibility of using more pillows or more supportive pillows, like the ones shaped like an inverted V. The aim is to raise your head and shoulders, not fold your body over at the waist. The practical problem is that most people move around a lot in their sleep, so maintaining a propped position for is difficult. But starting off the night in a tilted position might be helpful.

The other bit of advice sometimes given to those who suffer at night is to sleep on your left side and there is also some evidence to back this up.

The logic here is that your oesophagus takes a left turn before entering the stomach. So by lying on your left side, the final few centimetres of oesophagus slope downhill, encouraging any acid in your stomach to stay in its place. This is worth a try – but again, its probably impossible to stay in this position for long, once you are asleep. And of course it is not particularly easy to sleep propped up *and* on your side. But it is certainly worth experimenting to see if either of these help you get to sleep.

**Summary of chapter:**

- Try to find creative ways to reduce bending and lifting

- Practise methods of bending and lifting that bend the knees instead of the waist

- If you suffer at night:

- Have your last meal in the early evening

- Prop up the head of your bed.

- Or try sleeping on your left side

.

# Chapter 8

# Avoid Irritants

I mentioned earlier that if you are experiencing reflux symptoms it may be because there is inflammation in your oesophagus that has been caused by repeated acid reflux.

Inflammation is a wonderful thing that it will usually prevent a serious bacterial infection if you cut yourself. The trouble is that it doesn't just occur when you have a wound full of bacteria - other kinds of tissue damage can set it off, such as a sprained ankle, a burn, or acid damage. In those situations the inflammation itself can sometimes be damaging as there are lots of immune cells and chemicals in the area and instead of killing bacteria they may, if the inflammation is prolonged or frequent, damage some of the cells of the body.

Once you have a sore oesophagus, it would seem sensible to avoid things that are likely to further irritate it and delay healing. A good test is to imagine you have a sore eye. Some things, used in an eye-bath, would make it sting and get redder and if you rubbed your eye, you would inevitably slow the process of healing.

**So common sense would suggest:**

Don't swallow very hot drinks. A mouthful of fluid takes only a few seconds to travel through your oesophagus, which is not enough time to cool down. You don't want to add a heat burn to an existing acid burn and you certainly would not bathe your sore eye in hot coffee.

**It might also help to avoid:**

- Very acidic foods like lemon squash, grapefruit or pickles – if you had a sore eye you would not bathe it in vinegar

- Hot spices (chilli, ginger etc). Again the sore eye test tells us that these are likely to make your oesophagus more painful

- Abrasive food such as nuts, seeds, granola bars and dry toast unless you have chewed very thoroughly

While you are giving your oesophagus time to heal you could seek out smooth, bland foods like soup, pasta, yogurt, custard or ice cream.

There is no evidence that giving up a long list of foods reduces incidence of reflux. But individuals do report that particular foods make their symptoms worse. It could be that in some cases there is some mild, unnoticed inflammation of the oesophagus and a particular food irritates it further so that symptoms are noticed. It easy to imagine that a hot curry could tip the balance in this way. Or it could be that some foods irritate individual stomachs and cause them to be over-active, or encourage more of those brief relaxations of the LOS. We just don't know.

If you want to find out whether a particular food is to blame for *your* symptoms I suggest that you try to be scientific about it:

Try avoiding a single food for a week and keep a note of your symptoms every day. You give your symptoms 1-5 several times a day, perhaps and note it down.

Then eat the food for a couple of days and note your symptoms. Then cut the food out again and keep monitoring. A small experiment like this can help you to assess whether you are correct in your hunch that a particular food is better avoided.

The non-scientific approach would be to give up a whole list of foods, or to consume them in a random way making it difficult to nail down culprits. Once someone has suggested that chocolate may cause reflux, it is easy to point the finger of blame, whereas the real problem might have been the two hours of bending in the garden.

The advice to avoid peppermint is particularly mysterious when you consider that it is a popular ingredient in antacid medicines.

You may come across suggestions that you should avoid "acid foods" or eat an "alkaline diet" and so on. This is quite a popular concept in the world of alternative medicine (naturopaths, internet sites and so on) and is recommended freely for all kinds of conditions. For reflux sufferers this potentially creates confusion.

The idea is based on a new-age notion about "acid foods" that originated with Chinese categories of yin and yang. Under this system, meat and bread are classified as very acidic whereas lemons and grapes are considered alkaline. So when they say "acid" they don't mean acid at all. My advice is to steer clear of any therapists, books or websites that start talking about acid and alkaline foods or diets.

**Avoid alcohol**

If you had a sore eye, you wouldn't use an alcohol-based eyewash. It therefore stands to reason that if you have an inflamed oesophagus, bathing it in strong alcohol is not a good idea. The stronger the alcohol, the more it is likely to irritate an inflamed oesophagus. Spirits would sting anyone's eye, as would wine. So if you want a social drink that won't irritate your oesophagus, choose something very low in alcohol.

## Give up smoking

Or, better still, don't start. There seems to be an association between smoking and diseases of the oesophagus. Nicotine tends to relax internal muscles and may have an effect on the LOS. The ingredients of cigarettes are known to be carcinogenic.

## Burps and bubbles

Every time you swallow, a little air is taken down into your stomach. At times the LOS opens to allow some of the air to escape upwards. When the LOS opens and a bubble of air (a burp) travels back up, acid could escape with the air and cause more irritation. One of your *symptoms* might be frequent burping – air is escaping up through a weak valve.

Everyone burps but belching deliberately or forcefully might make your reflux symptoms worse.

Some people are quite talented belchers. They have got the knack of doing it on demand, sometimes quite loudly. They are using a combination of muscles to force out some air. I would suggest that if you suffer from reflux this is a bad idea.

You might also suffer from a vague feeling of fullness and discomfort that makes you wonder if you need to burp to relieve the pressure. If you have a habit of burping, try to resist the urge. And cut out that loud belching to impress your friends.

**Summary of chapter:**

If you are getting symptoms that suggest your oesophagus is sore or irritated, treat it kindly and think about what you are swallowing. And minimise burping and belching

.

# Chapter 9

# Reduce Stomach Activity

When there's food in your stomach, it's contracting frequently and quite forcefully to ensure that food particles are mixed with the chemicals of digestion. Its action is a lot like a washing machine, which agitates its contents to ensure that water and detergent reach all parts of the laundry. But instead of a rotary action, the stomach has a squeezing one. While your stomach is full and all this activity is taking place, acid is more likely to escape backwards. In fact there are medicines, sometimes prescribed for reflux (known as prokinetic drugs) that speed the passage of food through the stomach, with the aim of reducing the duration of stomach activity (see Chapter10 for more on medicines).

It stands to reason that the more hours in the day your stomach is busy digesting, the more active it will be and the more opportunities there are for reflux to occur.

**How can you adapt your eating habits to minimise stomach activity?**

The thing to remember is that your stomach works quite slowly. It takes about 3 to 4 hours, sometimes longer, to process a full meal and empty itself completely.

If you are swallowing large lumps of steak, that have not been well chewed, they will take a lot longer to digest than meat that has been minced or well-chewed. If you want to create less work for your stomach, chewing your food thoroughly could help.

High calorie foods, with lots of carbohydrates and fat, take longer to digest. So if you want a calmer stomach, eat things like low-fat natural yoghurt, egg, low fat cottage cheese, fruit and vegetables.

Reflux sufferers are often advised to eat smaller, more frequent meals. This could be worth a try, but you might find that eating frequently just keeps your stomach working all day long.

It could also encourage your stomach to adapt to smaller meals and thus further reduce your ability to eat a normal-sized meal without discomfort.

Logic would say eat moderately and avoid unusually big meals. Imagine you ate some bread, bacon and eggs for breakfast. A couple of hours later your stomach is starting to pass on this partly digested meal. Then you consume a large, full fat cappuccino and a blueberry muffin, keeping your stomach in action and depriving it of its rest period. If you want to allow your stomach its rest periods, it makes sense to avoiding snacks and high calorie drinks between meals. You will soon train your stomach to expect only three meals a day.

Alcohol may relax your stomach and slow digestion, which might be another reason why alcohol does not combine well with a tendency to reflux.

Some drugs, too, slow down the action of the digestive system. The most well known are opioids such as codeine.

Another time when the stomach churns is when it is expecting a meal, or one is overdue. It is probably also producing acid when this churning happens. So eating at regular times might help it to keep in a settled rhythm.

Emotion can affect the action of the stomach. During the second half of the 20th century there was a widely accepted medical belief that stress was *the* cause of stomach ulcers. This was based on research on rats that showed that if you subjected the poor animals to prolonged and quite severe stress they developed ulcers, along with a number of other serious conditions. These days the main cause of ulcers in humans is considered to be Helicobacter pylori, mentioned in Chapter 3 and the idea that gastric ailments are stress-related has become far less common. However an ulcer arising from stress is still a possibility. The digestive system can be affected by stress in many ways – loss of appetite; "butterflies in the stomach" due to stage fright; vomiting and diarrhoea caused by great fear or emotional shock, and so on. Depending on the kind of stress, and the individual, things can either speed up or slow down.

So it is not impossible that reflux in some people could be related to the churning effect of emotion on the stomach. If you experience frequent "butterflies in the stomach" this could be happening to you and you might benefit from some kind of stress management.

**Summary of chapter:**

Overloading your stomach will encourage it to be active for more of the time. Eat three meals a day at regular intervals and allow it to rest in between.

# Chapter 10

# Medicines and Self-Help

Self-help is not a quick fix. The suggestions in the previous chapters aren't going work miracles overnight. Many of them require persistence and effort. You need time to learn the breathing exercises and time to practise them before they strengthen your diaphragm. Improving your posture needs a change in established habits. So does changing the way you lift, bend and use the toilet. Losing weight definitely takes time.

Even the most determined self-helper needs to be patient.

We also know that putting up with the discomfort of reflux is not a good idea. Acid can cause damage and inflammation that doesn't necessarily heal overnight and can eventually contribute to cancer of the oesophagus.

There are a number of types of medicine that can help the symptoms of reflux. Some you can buy in the supermarket or pharmacy and others need a doctor's prescription. In this chapter I'll go through the various medicines, starting with the simple remedies that you can buy in a supermarket and progressing to those your doctor might prescribe. I will outline some of the advantages and disadvantages. I'll also consider whether it's a good idea to try alternative remedies such as herbs.

**Medicines for reflux**

**1. Alginates**

These are not drugs as such, because they are made from seaweed and don't interact with the cells or chemicals in your body. Neither are they herbal medicines. So side effects or interactions with prescription drugs are very unlikely. They work by creating a frothy layer that floats on top of the liquid in your stomach. This foamy barrier can prevent acid from leaking up into your oesophagus. Gaviscon is a well-known brand and supermarkets may sell their own brands. Products containing alginates often contain simple antacids and for this reason you should check the maximum dose.

**2. Antacids**

This word, meaning anti-acid, covers a range of medicines that reduce the acidity of in the oesophagus and stomach. They can be in the form of pills, powders, capsules, liquids or chewable tablets. Some can be bought over the counter and others are prescription drugs.

**2a. Simple antacids** have been around for a long time. They contain substances that react chemically with stomach acid and tend to neutralise it. They contain straightforward chemicals like calcium carbonate, aluminium hydroxide and magnesium hydroxide and can be bought without prescription. Examples are Rennies, Tums and Milk of Magnesia but there are many brands available. You may find that a local pharmacy or supermarket has a cheaper "own brand" that works just as well.

A single dose is probably not going to neutralise all your stomach contents if you have recently eaten. But it might reduce the acidity in your oesophagus enough to relieve a mild burning sensation.

It's best not to over-use these because excessive consumption can be harmful. Even calcium, a mineral that's very good for you in small amounts, can cause serious side effects if you consume too much. Refer to the instructions in the packaging for safe levels of use.

*If you are taking more and more antacid pills on a daily basis, you really need to see your doctor.* Also if you are taking any other medications, talk to your pharmacist (chemist) before self-medicating with antacids.

I don't recommend bicarbonate of soda (bicarb), or baking soda (same thing) for indigestion, despite the fact it is a traditional home remedy. A very simple chemical equation will reveal why:

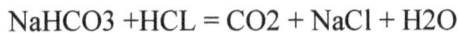

$$NaHCO_3 + HCL = CO_2 + NaCl + H_2O$$

Bicarbonate of soda reacts with hydrochloric acid (the acid found in the stomach) to produce carbon dioxide, sodium chloride (common salt) and water. The bicarbonate of soda will reduce the acidity in your oesophagus and stomach. The carbon dioxide produced will probably make you burp, which may feel like a result, but won't help. It is generally agreed that too much sodium chloride tends to raise blood pressure and for this reason I would not recommend anyone to take bicarb on a regular basis. People with certain serious medical conditions who have been advised to be on low sodium diets should avoid bicarbonate of soda. For healthy people it is OK to use bicarb as a one-off, if you don't have anything else in the house.

There are some branded products like Alka Seltzer that consist of bicarbonate of soda, citric acid and additives such as aspirin and caffeine. They are principally "hangover remedies" rather than indigestion treatments. The citric acid, when mixed with water, reacts chemically with the bicarb, causing a dramatic fizzing effect. This means that the b is already being changed into salt before you drink it, so it seems unlikely that it will have much of a soothing effect on acidity. I would not recommend these fizzy products for any kind of indigestion.

**2b Acid blockers** are modern drugs act in a very different way because they affect the cells in your stomach lining and reduce their acid output. This group of drugs is also used to treat some conditions in the stomach itself e.g. gastritis and ulcers. They are frequently prescribed by doctors and you may be able to buy lower dose versions in the pharmacy or supermarket.

*If you are taking more than one type of over the counter medicine at the same time, you should see your doctor.*

There are two main kinds of acid blockers:

- **H2-receptor blockers** were the first drugs to work in this way.

- **Proton pump inhibitors (PPIs)** block acid production much more effectively than H2 receptor-blockers and are now usually a doctor's first choice for reflux patients. They are currently the most popular prescribed drugs for oesophagitis and they are also given to gastritis sufferers. If you are prescribed these to heal an ulcer or suspected erosive oesophagitis you really should take the course.

## 3. Prokinetic medicines

If acid-blocking medicines fail to bring relief, your doctor may prescribe a prokinetic drug, which works by helping food pass more rapidly through your stomach. These can help in cases where stomach-emptying is not taking place at the normal pace. Diabetes and an overly-tight pyloric valve can be causes of slow emptying.

**What are the possible side effects of acid-blocking drugs?**

The production of stomach acid is normal, and if you prevent it, there may be some side effects. Side effects are not common but they will be listed on the leaflet inside the packaging. Government health advice does not recommend taking them continuously for the rest of your life, but many people do take them for years without ill effect.

NICE, the body that issues guidance to doctors in the UK, suggests a month or two of medication and then a break to see what happens. At the time of writing new guidelines are being prepared. The FDA, in the USA, recommends a 14-day course of treatment up to 3 times a year.

Apart from side effects there are some other reasons why it might be better to try to avoid long-term, continuous acid-blocking medication:

Anything that reduces the amount of acid in your stomach potentially affects the normal process of digestion. When there is less acid in the stomach it may make the digestion of some kinds of food e.g. meat and fish less effective.

There have been suggestions that this incomplete digestion of protein foods might cause food allergies but this may or may not be true.

Since stomach acid normally kills bacteria, acid-blockers can potentially increase your vulnerability to bacteria that cause vomiting or diarrhoea. There is some current concern that acid-blocking drugs are linked to increased incidence of Clostridium difficile infection. This is a particularly persistent form of diarrhoea, most often seen in weak hospital patients who have had a lot of antibiotics.

One study found that there seems to be a slightly increased risk of hip fracture in post-menopausal women who took PPIs for a long period *and who also smoked.*

It is important to be aware that stopping PPIs may cause a "rebound effect" in which your symptoms return when you stop the medicine. In a study of healthy individuals, with no prior reflux, symptoms developed when they took a short course of PPIs and then stopped them. This is concerning because it means that it may be hard to "come off" PPIs once you have started. If you take a course of PPIs and reflux comes back when you stop, just wait and see what happens after two or three of weeks.

Drug interactions can occur between antacids and other medicines and acid-blocking drugs can interfere with the body's ability to absorb another drug.

*Check with your doctor or pharmacist if you are on any prescription drug and add an acid-blocker to the mix.*

Having said all that, these drugs are considered extremely safe and large numbers of people take them for long periods with no harmful effects.

You should also be aware that several types of prescription medicines, given for other conditions, can contribute to reflux. If you have recently changed your medication and started to have reflux, make an appointment and discuss this with your doctor.

*Don't stop taking any prescribed medication without talking to your doctor.*

**Medicines recap for shoppers**

In my local supermarkets and pharmacies there is a bewildering array of indigestion remedies with various combinations of ingredients. I recommend that you read the labels carefully and check what you are buying. Here is a quick summary of the ingredients you will come across in that small print:

**Alginates** – found in liquids and tablets. Create a foamy layer in stomach. Very safe. Often mixed with a simple antacid. Gaviscon is a well-known brand but there are others.

**Calcium carbonate** – a simple acid-neutralising chemical. Safe unless you take a lot.

**Bicarbonate of Soda/ sodium bicarbonate** – will neutralise stomach acid and make you burp, but will also increase your salt (sodium) intake.

**Magnesium hydroxide** – the active ingredient of Milk of Magnesia. This product has been around for well over 100 years. It's an antacid and a laxative. So don't take it if you have diarrhoea, even if your granny gave it to you for every kind of tummy upset.

**Bismuth** – the key ingredient of Pepto-bismol, another product that has been around for over a century. Originally a treatment for diarrhoea, it can cause constipation. Not an acid neutralizer so I would not recommend it for reflux symptoms.

**Salicylates or salicylic acid** are names for aspirin. Found in Alka Seltzer, Pepto-bismol and other products. Not recommended for those with a tendency to gastritis as it can irritate the stomach lining and increase the chance of bleeding. Aspirin is not suitable for children.

**Ranitidine** – an H2-receptor blocker. Will reduce acid production. Zantac is a common brand but around the world it is sold under many names.

**Omeprazole** – this is a proton pump inhibitor and will block acid production. If it is on sale it may be a lower dose than a prescription dose. There are several other PPIs but this seems to be the most common. You might also see it described as Losec, Prilosec, Losepine and many other names around the world.

If you are not sure about any medicine ingredients and whether they are suitable for you, or if you want anything explained, ask a qualified pharmacist. This is one of the advantages of buying from a local pharmacy, not an online company. Drugs bought over the Internet may be cheap but they may not always be of good quality.

And do read the labels, and the advice on the leaflets inside.

**What kind of patient are you?**

I've noticed there are several types of people when it comes to attitudes to doctors and medicine.

**1.The Brave**

They don't want to bother the doctor and tend to struggle on alone. They may believe that suffering by choice is a sign of virtue. They tend to say "Don't fuss, it's nothing".

**2. The Ostrich**

Similar to the Brave but their reason for avoiding the doctor is that they fear bad news and "would rather not know" so they dismiss their symptoms and try not to think about them.

**3. The New-Age Warrior**

Believes the drugs doctors give out are dangerous and unnatural. Anything that looks "alternative" must be a better option. Convinced they can beat illness with the help of herbs and beautiful thoughts.

### 4. The Professional Patient

Likes going to the doctor and follows medical advice diligently. Loves to talk about their ailments.

### 5. The Helpless

Expects doctors to solve all medical problems with a prescription and doesn't see why they should give up smoking/ lose weight or change their lives in any way.

The first three have a tendency to avoid taking medication and the danger is that they will do so when medication is a really good idea. Numbers 4 and 5 might have a tendency to become over-dependent on medication.

Most of us will have one or other of these tendencies but there is a sixth category – the Independent. You inform yourself about health issues, you go to the doctor if you think your symptoms might be worrying, you'd prefer not to take long-term medication if possible and you try to take responsibility for keeping healthy.

But just in case you are in any doubt, my position is: if you have persistent "indigestion", or any digestive symptoms that come on suddenly, see your doctor (see Chapter 3). Don't forget to discuss whether your reflux could be a side-effect of any other medicines you are taking or whether any drugs prescribed are safe to take alongside any other medication.

If your doctor agrees that you have reflux you will probably be offered acid-controlling drugs.

At this point you could ask if you could go away and try using non-prescription medicine while you work on self-help.

Or

You could take the course of prescription drugs while starting to work on your self-help. Then, with your doctor's agreement, try a couple of weeks off the medication to see how much your symptoms have improved.

It depends on how severe your symptoms are, and whether you have already tried over the counter medicines.

When considering whether or not to take acid blocking drugs, and for how long, don't be a martyr because, for some people, PPIs are essential to prevent ulceration or long-term damage. It may be that you will always need some help from some kind of medicine, but until you have tried helping yourself you won't know if this is the case.

**Herbs**

I would not advise taking any herbal medicines without first checking with your doctor for a diagnosis and checking with your doctor that the herbs are a safe mix with any other medicines you are taking.

The things to bear in mind with herbs are:

- If a substance has a real effect on the way the body works, it could have some side effects

- A herb may interact with other medicines (increasing or decreasing their effect)

- If it does not have a real effect on the body, it's a waste of money

- Herbs are not produced in a standard way with standard strength and measured dosages

- Herbs have not been safety tested in the same way as prescription medicines

- Products could be contaminated, or contain something other than the substance you think you are buying

If you are determined to try herbal medicines I suggest buying them from a retailer, governed by the laws of your country about the safety and description of medicines. Never buy them via the Internet because you have no way of knowing if the product is safe, or even if it contains the substance described on the label. There are thousands of frauds on the Internet that exploit people who are unwell or even seriously ill.

These comments also apply to Chinese and Ayurvedic medicines, which are mainly based on herbs.

Of course there are lots of harmless herbs used for cooking in small quantities are not known for having an effect on the workings of the body.

**Surgery**

Finally I should mention that there are surgical techniques that have been used to alleviate reflux (including hernia surgery). These are aimed at tightening up the LOS.

The notion of having a quick operation to cure reflux may sound appealing. If you have to pay for a prescription drugs you may feel that it is more cost-effective to have an operation than pay for medicine for years. But there are some things you should consider if surgery is suggested.

Surgery always carries risks. If you took a large group of healthy individuals, gave them a general anaesthetic and opened up their abdomens, had a brief look around and stitched them up again, a small percentage would develop life-threatening post-operative complications such as blood loss, infection, pneumonia, blood clots on the lungs and many others. There is also the risk that an operation will fail to cure your reflux or that it might cause side effects. If you are offered an operation I would suggest that you quiz the surgeon about success statistics, rates of complications and side effects before making a decision.

Before deciding on surgery, many surgeons would advise that your try self-help first and tell you to lose weight, cut right down on alcohol and cut out smoking. Whether or not giving up smoking reduces your reflux, surgeons always prefer operating on non-smokers as there are fewer complications. They would also question whether your reflux couldn't be controlled by high dose PPIs.

When assessing whether you are a suitable candidate for surgery they may also consider whether you are suffering from "volume reflux" (acid gushing up into your throat or mouth) at night as this indicates you have little in the way of an anti-reflux barrier. For some people, with severe symptoms, an operation can be the only way to bring them the relief they need.

**Summary of chapter:**

Alginates and simple antacids: very unlikely to have side effects unless you exceed recommended limits. Can be used as required for relief of mild symptoms. Check with your pharmacist if you are taking other medicines.

Acid blockers: stop acid production in the cells that line the stomach. This could have side effects. They need to be taken daily. There could be a rebound effect when you stop which could create dependency.

Anti-kinetics: recommended by doctors for cases where other drugs don't work.

Herbs: untested and unproven. Doses not regulated. Could be contaminated.

Surgery is needed in some cases but does have risks

**Final reminder:**

If you have sudden-onset, frequent, severe or persistent pain, see a doctor and take advice. You should be checked for serious conditions such as ulcers. People can die of stomach ulcers if they eat into blood vessels or make a hole through the stomach wall. These cannot be treated by any form of alternative practitioner, self-help or over the counter medicines.

# Chapter 11

## How to Help Yourself

I have previously outlined some of the possible long-term consequences of reflux (in Chapter 3) and the risk of these should not be taken lightly. But if you take action and keep your symptoms under control, you can avoid these. Self-help alone might enable you to control your reflux, or you might need a combination of self-help and medication. But by reading this book you have armed yourself with the information you need.

Each of us has our own combination of physical and lifestyle factors that combine to produce symptoms. The causes of reflux are "multifactorial" and only you can assess which factors are likely to be contributing in your case.

In some, excess abdominal fat is the key factor. In others, it's a job that involves too much sitting or a lot of lifting. Many people have a weak diaphragm that never gets a work-out and poor posture is extremely common. In some people a hiatus hernia is a contributing cause – but remember that not all those with a weak hiatus have reflux symptoms.

Some people can clear up their symptoms simply easily. Others have an inefficient LOS and will always have to nurse it along by maximizing the strength of their diaphragm and managing the way they bend and lift. Some can never completely eliminate their symptoms and for them, self-help means minimising the amount of medication or avoiding the need for surgery.

The best way for you to manage your reflux should be tailored to reflect your body, your lifestyle and your preferences.

There are lots of suggestions in this book about ways to reduce your symptoms. None of them will require a financial outlay but many of them require some focus, work and persistence on your part.

You may have tried some of them already. You'd have to be really committed to try them *all* at once and I don't recommend this. Not unless you're the kind of person who can make ten New Year's resolutions and stick to them all!

I suggest that you don't try to change too many things at once.

But you may be wondering where to start.

Only *you* know the extent of your symptoms and only *you* know your own starting point. You may have previously learned deep breathing techniques, you may have excellent posture and you may have a weight problem – or none of these may apply. No single plan would suit everyone. So start by picking one or two areas that make sense to you and start working on those.

**Here is a reminder of my main suggestions:**

- Lose some weight to reduce fat around your waist

- Strengthen your diaphragm with breathing exercises

- Don't wear clothes that squash your waist or abdomen

- Take moderate exercise, such as a daily brisk walk

- If you are more active, exercise without straining or squashing your abdomen

- Train yourself to sit with a more upright posture

- Practise better ways of bending and lifting

- Don't strain on the toilet or when lifting

- Avoid constipation by eating a high fibre diet

- Avoid constipation by adopting regular habits

- Don't swallow irritating foods

- Don't deliberately belch

- Don't eat huge meals

- Eat your last meal of the day early in the evening

- Prop up you shoulders when you go to bed

- Let your stomach have regular rest periods during the day

While you are working on your chosen areas you may be able to control your symptoms with over-the-counter remedies. If light self-medication doesn't work, try acid-blocking prescription drugs for a short period. Then stop for a few weeks and see how you get on. Remember there can be a "rebound effect" when you stop taking these drugs and it may take a while to settle. My personal priorities continue to be the diaphragm exercises, working on my posture (particularly at my desk) and avoiding bending from the waist. I'm also trying to get rid of a couple of kilos of "spare tyre" around my waist.

If you have fat around your waist, particularly if is giving you a bulging "paunch", I would strongly suggest that its reduction it should be high on your list of priorities. This may not appeal to you, but it is important for the health of your oesophagus, as well as for several other aspects of health.

Whatever you choose, set yourself some simple, achievable goals. It's best to avoid vague and negative goals like "I will stop eating things that are bad for me" or "I will give up bending". Instead make your goals *positive*, short term and relatively easy to achieve, such as:

- I will eat oats for breakfast

- I will eat a large portion of vegetables every evening

- I will practise breathing exercises during the TV advertisement breaks

It takes at least a couple of weeks to change a habit. You have to keep reminding yourself and shrugging off the occasional mistake. If you have ever moved house in the same town, you may well have automatically driven back to your old address, as I did recently. Don't worry about your lapses – they will get less frequent with time. The first step is to build up your awareness of how you move, how you sit, how you breathe, how you eat and how you use the toilet. In the mornings, when I feel a little stiff, I am often tempted to bend from the waist rather than bend my knees. But the incentive of being free of discomfort and being able to enjoy life more, keeps me motivated.

As a final incentive to change, I'd like to point out that many of the suggestions in this book have additional positive benefits that act as extra rewards your efforts.

- Losing weight helps you to feel more comfortable and will reduce your risk of developing a long list of diseases, from diabetes to worn-out joints

- Cutting out snacks between meals and in the evening can help you to control your weight

- Eating a high-fibre diet is much the best thing for your bowels

- A daily walk has numerous health benefits and can also help to lift your mood

- Improving your posture will strengthen your back muscles and make you look, taller, slimmer and more confident

- If you strengthen your legs by using them to bend and lift you'll be steadier on your feet and have a spring in your step

- Working on your diaphragm may improve your lung capacity for other activities, such as singing and swimming

- Slow, deep breathing is also an effective way of controlling anxiety

- Oh – and if you are spending money on medicines, less need for them will save you money

Finally I'd like to wish you well with your self-help plans. Your body is an incredibly complex, largely self-maintaining organism. Most of its systems run happily with no requirements beyond a supply of food, water and oxygen. There are a few though, that benefit from a bit of regular maintenance. Treat them well and they will continue to give good service for years to come.

# Appendix

# How the digestive system works

This section is for readers who want a quick recap of how the digestive system works.

Food is ingested when it is eaten, digested when it is broken down into a useable form and absorbed when it enters the bloodstream.

Food consists of three main groups of chemicals: proteins, carbohydrates and fats. The molecules involved are large and complex, unlike the simple molecules such as H2O and CO2 that you may remember from school science. A molecule of water contains just 3 atoms but a protein molecule may contain thousands of atoms. These large food molecules must be broken down into much smaller molecules before they can pass through the walls of the intestines and enter the blood stream so they can be used.

There are also tiny amounts of vitamins and minerals in food. These do not need to be broken down by digestion. Also food contains a lot of water.

The food is broken down in two ways:

## 1. Mechanical

Lumps of food are chewed in the mouth to mash them up and begin the process of breaking food down into tiny particles. The muscular action of the stomach also helps to break it up. Imagine you had a plastic bag full of well-cooked peas and some water. If you shook the bag for five minutes the peas would start to disintegrate. This is what happens to food in the stomach. The particles need to be broken down until they are about 2 mm across before they are moved on.

## 2. Chemical

Imagine that the food molecules are like elaborate necklaces with hundreds of interwoven beads. The action of digestive chemicals breaks the necklaces apart into short fragments – simpler molecules. All carbohydrates and sugars are broken down into glucose molecules. Proteins are broken down into amino acid molecules. Fats are broken down into smaller molecules as well.

The main chemicals that do this work are enzymes. They act like scissors, snipping the big molecules into smaller and smaller pieces. Some enzymes work on proteins, others on carbohydrates or fats.

Stomach acid is another chemical that helps to break down some foods. It acts like a marinade on lumps of meat and fish, softening them up and starting to break them apart, so that the enzymes can do their work more easily. If you have ever taken a bit of raw fish and put it in lemon juice you will have seen the dramatic change that acid can cause. (Salmon works best for this experiment as the dark orange flesh turns pale pink and more opaque. In fact it looks like cooked salmon.)

The enzymes and acid are produced by the glands that line the digestive system. Large quantities of digestive juices are produced every day – quite a lot of saliva, a couple of litres of gastric juice (produced in the stomach) and several additional litres by the gall bladder and intestines.

This fluid is needed because the enzymes only work in a liquid bath. Some enzymes work well in an acidic liquid while others work well in an alkaline environment. The excess water is re-absorbed by the colon.

As each stage of digestion is completed, the food is passed on by the muscular squeezing known as peristalsis.

The walls of the digestive system contain a complicated system of nerve cells and these are able to sense the progress of digestion and control the whole process.

**Stage by stage:**

1. In the mouth food is chewed and mixed with saliva, which contains a digestive enzyme that starts to break down starch.

2. In the stomach the food is mixed with acidic gastric juice, which contains the enzyme pepsin that starts to break down proteins. This phase lasts 2-4 hours.

3. In the first section of the small intestine food breakdown is completed. The liver and the pancreas work with the glands in the walls of the intestine to produce all the chemicals needed. Pancreatic juices neutralize the stomach acid and bile from the liver (via the gall bladder) breaks up fat droplets much like a detergent does when you wash up oily pans.

4. In the lower end of the small intestine most of the absorption of food molecules takes place. Its lining is folded into finger-shaped villi, which give it a very large surface area.

5. In the colon (bowel, or large intestine) "friendly" gut bacteria extract some additional nutrients from dietary fibre. The colon then absorbs most of the water and forms the faeces, which are stored at its lower end. This absorption of water is essential. It must to returned to circulation in the blood. In diarrhoea everything goes through the colon far too quickly and water is lost rapidly from the body causing dehydration. Treatment of severe cases often involves making sure that the body is kept hydrated while the illness runs its course.

# References

## Chapter 1 Symptoms and sufferers

Ness-Jensen E, Lindam A, Lagergren J, Hveem K. Changes in prevalence, incidence and spontaneous loss of gastro-oesophageal reflux symptoms: a prospective population-based cohort study, the HUNT study.

*Gut* 2012 Oct ;61(10):1390-7.

Boeckxstaens G, Hashem B, El-Serag BH, Smout AJPM, Kahrilas PJ

Symptomatic reflux disease: the present, the past and the future *Gut* 2014 Jul;63(7):1185-93

## Chapter 2 - Why reflux happens

Joliffe D. M. Practical gastric physiology *Contin Educ Anaesth Crit Care Pain* (2009) 9 (6): 173-177.

Barry D.W. and Vaezi M.F Laryngopharyngeal reflux: More questions than answers *Cleveland Clinic Journal of Medicine* 2010 May; 77 (5): 327-334

Dent J, Dodds WJ, Friedman RH, Sekiguchi T, Hogan WJ, Arndorfer RC, Petrie DJ. Mechanism of gastroesophageal reflux in recumbent asymptomatic human subjects. *J Clin Invest.* 1980 Feb; 65(2):256-67.

Bombeck CT, Dillard DH, Nyhus LM Muscular Anatomy of the Gastroeosophageal Junction and Role of the Phrenoesophageal Ligament, Autopsy study of Sphincter Mechanism *Annals of Surgery* 1966 Oct; 643 - 652

**Chapter 3 Words of Warning**

Navarro Silvera SA, Mayne ST, Gammon MD, Vaughan TL, Chow WH, Dubin JA, Dubrow R, Stanford JL, West AB, Rotterdam H, Blot WJ, Risch HA. Diet and lifestyle factors and risk of subtypes of esophageal and gastric cancers: classification tree analysis. *Ann Epidemiol.* 2014 Jan; 24(1):50-7.

Shefalee Loth

Had dodgy advice from a nutritional therapist? We have!

*Which website*, http://www.which.co.uk 16 January 2012

**Chapter 4 – Self-Help Strategies**

Ness-Jensen E, Lindam A, Lagergren J and Hveem K Tobacco Smoking Cessation and Improved Gastroesophageal Reflux: A Prospective Population-Based Cohort Study: The HUNT Study. *The American Journal of Gastroenterology* 2014 Feb; 109, 171-177

Kaltenbach T, Crockett S, Gerson LB. Are lifestyle measures effective in patients with gastroesophageal reflux disease? An evidence-based approach.

*Arch Intern Med.* 2006 May 8;166(9):965-71.

Gerson L.B. The Effects of Lifestyle Modifications on GERD *Gastroenterol Hepatol (N Y)* 2009 Sep; 5(9): 613–615.

**Chapter 5 Strengthen your Diaphragm**

R K Mittal, D F Rochester, and R W McCallum Effect of the diaphragmatic contraction on lower oesophageal sphincter pressure in man. *Gut* 1987 Dec; 28(12): 1564–1568

Eherer A.J., Netolitzky F, Hogenauer C, Puschnig G, Hinterleitner TA, Scheidl S, Kraxner W, Keris GJ, Hoffman KM Positive effect of abdominal breathing exercise on gastroesphageal reflux disease: a randomized, controlled study.

*Am J Gastroenterol.* Mar 2012, 107(3);372-8

Eherer A Management of gastroesophageal reflux disease: lifestyle modification and alternative approaches. *Dig Dis.* 2014;32 (1-2)149-51

Pickering M, Jones JFX The diaphragm: two physiological muscles in one

*J Anat.* Oct 2002; 201(4): 305–312.

Lindgren H Gord Treatment without drugs
http://www.hanslindgren.com/blog/gord-treatment-without-drugs/

Bitnar et al Crural Diaphragm Function Monitoring in the Lower Esophageal Sphincter Area. http://www.rehabps.cz/data/Bitnar.pdf

**Chapter 6 Reduce Pressure**

Collings K.L., Pierce P. F., Rodriguez-Stanley S., Bemben M., Miner P.B.

Esophageal reflux in conditioned runners, cyclists, and weightlifters. *Med Sci Sports Exerc.* 2003 May;35(5):730-5.

Maddison KJ, Shepherd KL, Hillman DR, Eastwood PR. Function of the lower esophageal sphincter during and after high-intensity exercise.*Med Sci Sports Exerc.* 2005 Oct;37(10):1728-33.

Jacobson BC, Somers SC, Fuchs CS, Kelly CP, Camargo CA., Jr Body-mass index and symptoms of gastroesophageal reflux in women. *N Engl J Med.* 2006; 354:2340–2348

Festi D1, Scaioli E, Baldi F, Vestito A, Pasqui F, Di Biase AR, Colecchia A.

Body weight, lifestyle, dietary habits and gastroesophageal reflux disease *World J Gastroenterol.* 2009 Apr;15 (14):1690-701.

El-Serag HB, Ergun GA, Pandolfino J, Fitzgerald S, Tran T, Kramer JR.

Obesity increases oesophageal acid exposure. *Gut* 2007;56:749–755.

Ness-Jensen E, Lindam A, Lagergren J, Hveem K. Weight loss and reduction in gastroesophageal reflux. A prospective population-based cohort study: the HUNT study. *Am J Gastroenterol.* 2013 Mar;108(3):376-82.

Shafik A, Shafik A.A., Sibai O.E. and Mostafa R.M. Effect of straining on diaphragmatic crura with identification of the straining-crural reflex. The "reflex theory" in gastroesophageal competence. *BMC Gastroenterology* 2004, 4:24

## Chapter 7 Work with gravity

Kaltenbach T, Crockett S, Gerson LB. Are lifestyle measures effective in patients with gastroesophageal reflux disease? An evidence-based approach.*Arch Intern Med.* 2006 May 8;166(9):965-71.

Gerson L.B. The Effects of Lifestyle Modifications on GERD *Gastroenterol Hepatol (N Y).* 2009 Sep; 5(9): 613–615.

## Chapter 10 Medicines and Self-Help

Khalili H, Huang E S, Jacobson B. C., Camargo C.A., Feskanich D, Chan A.T.

Use of proton pump inhibitors and risk of hip fracture in relation to dietary and lifestyle factors: a prospective cohort study *BMJ* 2012; 344

Deshpande A, Pant C, Pasupuleti V, Rolston DD, Jain A, Deshpande N, Thota P, Sferra TJ, Hernandez AV. Association between proton pump inhibitor therapy and Clostridium difficile infection in a meta-analysis. *Clin Gastroenterol Hepatol.* 2012 Mar;10(3):225-33.

Reimer C, et al "Proton-pump inhibitor therapy induces acid-related symptoms in healthy volunteers after withdrawal of therapy" *Gastroenterology* 2009; 137: 80-87.

McColl KEL, Gillen D "Evidence that proton-pump inhibitor therapy induces the symptoms it is used to treat" *Gastroenterology* 2009; 137: 20-22.

# Information sources on the Internet

Always use reputable websites, rather than those who have a vested interest in selling supplements or those who are pushing a particular agenda.

**Health on the Net** http://www.hon.ch/ is a site that helps to filter out disreputable sites.

Information found on forums or on "ask a question" website should not be viewed as reliable. This is also true of many newspaper and magazine articles, which often blend a pinch of science with the opinions of alternative practitioners. Assume articles are written by journalists without a medical or scientific background unless there is evidence to the contrary.

**Cochrane Collaboration** reviews – a good source of independent reviews on health topics by scientists who give their time freely. The reviewers filter out poorly designed studies and assess well-conducted research. Particularly useful if you are thinking of trying any alternative/complementary treatments. http://www2.cochrane.org/reviews/

**NHS Choices:** UK government advice on health and wide range of diseases and health issues. Comprehensive and clear. http://www.nhs.uk/

The NHS has an evidence portal that can be a good place to find medical articles http://www.evidence.nhs.uk/

**UK Medicines and Healthcare Products Regulatory Agency** (MHRA)

Regulates the sale and use of prescription and herbal drugs. Site contains advice about the use of herbal medicine and specific warnings about herbal products that have been found to be contaminated or unsafe. http://www.mhra.gov.uk

**NHS National Institute for Health and Clinical Excellence (NICE)**

National guidelines on the use of drugs and other treatments within UK health system. http://www.nice.org.uk/

This website is run by UK family doctors to provide non-medical people with good quality information: http://www.patient.co.uk

**And in the USA:**

Healthfinder.gov, a U.S. Government health education site

http://www.healthfinder.gov

**Medline Plus** is a U.S. government-funded health advice site

http://www.nlm.nih.gov/medlineplus/

**U. S. Food and Drugs Administration (FDA)** Is the licensing body for medicines in the USA. It contains information about health protection, drugs, supplements, foods and a wide range of health-related topics.

http://www.fda.gov/

Many countries have their own equivalent websites with specific advice about national vaccination schedules, specific disease risks, local parasites etc.

Larger charities often have useful patient information on their websites. Note that charities may be receiving large donations from drug companies and may overstate the benefits of latest expensive medicines.

If you want to look at information about cancer of the oesophagus or other cancer-related information I find that Cancer Research UK has good site. http://www.cancerresearchuk.org

# Also by Jessica Madge:

Your Intelligent Immune System (2012)

**To stay in touch with the author:**

Visit her author site on:

**http://www.amazon.co.uk/Jessica-Madge**

Follow her on Twitter **@jess_madge**

Blogs: **http://jessica-madge.blogspot.co.uk**

**http://appealingtoreasonblog.blogspot.co.uk**

*9 780095 749515 9*